Medifocus Guidebook on:

Non-Hodgkin's Lymphoma

Last Update: 02 February 2012

Medifocus.com, Inc.

**11529 Daffodil Lane
Suite 200
Silver Spring, MD 20902**

www.medifocus.com

(800) 965-3002

MediFocus Guide #HM009

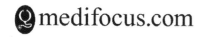

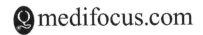

How To Use This Medifocus Guidebook

Before you start to review your *Guidebook*, it would be helpful to familiarize yourself with the organization and content of the information that is included in the Guidebook. Your *MediFocus Guidebook* is organized into the following five major sections.

- **Section 1: Background Information** - This section provides detailed information about the organization and content of the *Guidebook* including tips and suggestions for conducting additional research about the condition.

- **Section 2: The Intelligent Patient Overview** - This section is a comprehensive overview of the condition and includes important information about the cause of the disease, signs and symptoms, how the condition is diagnosed, the treatment options, quality of life issues, and questions to ask your doctor.

- **Section 3: Guide to the Medical Literature** - This section opens the door to the latest cutting-edge research and clinical advances recently published in leading medical journals. It consists of an extensive, focused selection of journal article references with links to the PubMed abstracts (summaries) of the articles. PubMed is the U.S. National Library of Medicine's database of references and abstracts from more than 4,500 medical and scientific articles published worldwide.

- **Section 4: Centers of Research** - This section is a unique directory of doctors, researchers, hospitals, medical centers, and research institutions with specialized interest and, in many cases, clinical expertise in the management of patients with the condition. You can use the "Centers of Research" directory to contact, consults, or network with leading experts in the field and to locate a hospital or medical center that can help you.

- **Section 5: Tips for Finding and Choosing a Doctor** - This section of your *Guidebook* offers important tips for how to find physicians as well as suggestions for how to make informed choices about choosing a doctor who is right for you.

- **Section 6: Directory of Organizations** - This section of your *Guidebook* is a directory of select disease organizations and support groups that are in the business of helping patients and their families by providing access to information, resources, and services. Many of these organizations can answer your questions, enable you to network with other patients, and help you find a doctor in your geographical area who specializes in managing your condition.

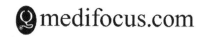

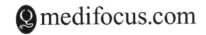 medifocus.com

Disclaimer

Medifocus.com, Inc. serves only as a clearinghouse for medical health information and does not directly or indirectly practice medicine. Any information provided by *Medifocus.com, Inc.* is intended solely for educating our clients and should not be construed as medical advice or guidance, which should always be obtained from a licensed physician or other health-care professional. As such, the client assumes full responsibility for the appropriate use of the medical and health information contained in the Guidebook and agrees to hold *Medifocus.com, Inc.* and any of its third-party providers harmless from any and all claims or actions arising from the clients' use or reliance on the information contained in this Guidebook. Although *Medifocus.com, Inc.* makes every reasonable attempt to conduct a thorough search of the published medical literature, the possibility always exists that some significant articles may be missed.

Copyright

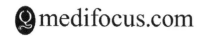

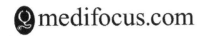
Table of Contents

Background Information 9
   Introduction 9
   About Your Medifocus Guidebook 11
   Ordering Full-Text Articles 15

The Intelligent Patient Overview 19

Guide to the Medical Literature 61
   Introduction 61
   Recent Literature: What Your Doctor Reads 63
      Review Articles 63
      General Interest Articles 83
      Drug Therapy Articles 100
      Clinical Trials Articles 107
      Radiation Therapy Articles 132
      Stem Cell Transplantation Articles 133
      Radioimmunotherapy Articles 138

Centers of Research 143
   United States 145
   Other Countries 163

Tips on Finding and Choosing a Doctor 183

Directory of Organizations 193

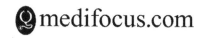

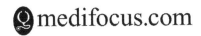medifocus.com

1 - Background Information

Introduction

Chronic or life-threatening illnesses can have a devastating impact on both the patient and the family. In today's new world of medicine, many consumers have come to realize that they are the ones who are primarily responsible for their own health care as well as for the health care of their loved ones.

When facing a chronic or life-threatening illness, you need to become an educated consumer in order to make an informed health care decision. Essentially that means finding out everything about the illness - the treatment options, the doctors, and the hospitals - so that you can become an educated health care consumer and make the tough decisions. In the past, consumers would go to a library and read everything available about a particular illness or medical condition. In today's world, many turn to the Internet for their medical information needs.

The first sites visited are usually the well known health "portals" or disease organizations and support groups which contain a general overview of the condition for the layperson. That's a good start but soon all of the basic information is exhausted and the need for more advanced information still exists. What are the latest "cutting-edge" treatment options? What are the results of the most up-to-date clinical trials? Who are the most notable experts? Where are the top-ranked medical institutions and hospitals?

The best source for authoritative medical information in the United States is the National Library of Medicine's medical database called PubMed, that indexes citations and abstracts (brief summaries) of over 7 million articles from more than 3,800 medical journals published worldwide. PubMed was developed for medical professionals and is the primary source utilized by health care providers for keeping up with the latest advances in clinical medicine.

A typical PubMed search for a specific disease or condition, however, usually retrieves hundreds or even thousands of "hits" of journal article citations. That's an avalanche of information that needs to be evaluated and transformed into truly useful knowledge. What are the most relevant journal articles? Which ones apply to your specific situation? Which articles are considered to be the most authoritative - the ones your physician would rely on in making clinical decisions? This is where *Medifocus.com* provides an effective solution.

Medifocus.com has developed an extensive library of *MediFocus Guidebooks* covering a wide spectrum of chronic and life threatening diseases. Each *MediFocus Guidebook* is a high quality, up- to-date digest of "professional-level" medical information consisting of the most relevant citations and abstracts of journal articles published in authoritative, trustworthy medical journals. This information represents the latest advances known to modern medicine for the treatment and management of the condition, including published results from clinical trials. Each *Guidebook* also includes a valuable index of leading authors and medical institutions as well as a directory of disease organizations and support groups. *MediFocus Guidebooks* are reviewed, revised and updated every 4-months to ensure that you receive the latest and most up-to-date information about the specific condition.

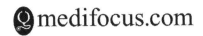medifocus.com

About Your MediFocus Guidebook

Introduction

Your *MediFocus Guidebook* is a valuable resource that represents a comprehensive synthesis of the most up-to-date, advanced medical information published about the condition in well-respected, trustworthy medical journals. It is the same type of professional-level information used by physicians and other health-care professionals to keep abreast of the latest developments in biomedical research and clinical medicine. The *Guidebook* is intended for patients who have a need for more advanced, in-depth medical information than is generally available to consumers from a variety of other resources. The primary goal of a *MediFocus Guidebook* is to educate patients and their families about their treatment options so that they can make informed health-care decisions and become active participants in the medical decision making process.

The *Guidebook* production process involves a team of experienced medical research professionals with vast experience in researching the published medical literature. This team approach to the development and production of the *MediFocus Guidebooks* is designed to ensure the accuracy, completeness, and clinical relevance of the information. The *Guidebook* is intended to serve as a basis for a more meaningful discussion between patients and their health-care providers in a joint effort to seek the most appropriate course of treatment for the disease.

Guidebook Organization and Content

Section 1 - Background Information
This section provides detailed information about the organization and content of the *Guidebook* including tips and suggestions for conducting additional research about the condition.

Section 2 - The Intelligent Patient Overview
This section of your *MediFocus Guidebook* represents a detailed overview of the disease or condition specifically written from the patient's perspective. It is designed to satisfy the basic informational needs of consumers and their families who are confronted with the illness and are facing difficult choices. Important aspects which are addressed in "The Intelligent Patient" section include:

- The etiology or cause of the disease
- Signs and symptoms
- How the condition is diagnosed

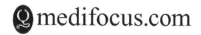 **medifocus.com**

- The current standard of care for the disease
- Treatment options
- New developments
- Important questions to ask your health care provider

Section 3 - Guide to the Medical Literature

This is a roadmap to important and up-to-date medical literature published about the condition from authoritative, trustworthy medical journals. This is the same information that is used by physicians and researchers to keep up with the latest developments and breakthroughs in clinical medicine and biomedical research. A broad spectrum of articles is included in each *MediFocus Guidebook* to provide information about standard treatments, treatment options, new clinical developments, and advances in research. To facilitate your review and analysis of this information, the articles are grouped by specific categories. A typical *MediFocus Guidebook* usually contains one or more of the following article groupings:

- *Review Articles:* Articles included in this category are broad in scope and are intended to provide the reader with a detailed overview of the condition including such important aspects as its cause, diagnosis, treatment, and new advances.

- *General Interest Articles:* These articles are broad in scope and contain supplementary information about the condition that may be of interest to select groups of patients.

- *Drug Therapy:* Articles that provide information about the effectiveness of specific drugs or other biological agents for the treatment of the condition.

- *Surgical Therapy:* Articles that provide information about specific surgical treatments for the condition.

- *Clinical Trials:* Articles in this category summarize studies which compare the safety and efficacy of a new, experimental treatment modality to currently available standard treatments for the condition. In many cases, clinical trials represent the latest advances in the field and may be considered as being on the "cutting edge" of medicine. Some of these experimental treatments may have already been incorporated into clinical practice.

The following information is provided for each of the articles referenced in this section of your *MediFocus Guidebook:*

- Article title

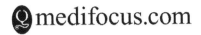

- Author Name(s)
- Institution where the study was done
- Journal reference (Volume, page numbers, year of publication)
- Link to Abstract (brief summary of the actual article)

Linking to Abstracts: Most of the medical journal articles referenced in this section of your *MediFocus Guidebook* include an abstract (brief summary of the actual article) that can be accessed online via the National Library of Medicine's PubMed® database. You can easily access the individual article abstracts online by entering the individual URL address for a particular article into your web browser, or by going to the URL listed on the bottom of each page of this section.

Section 4 - Centers of Research

We've compiled a unique directory of doctors, researchers, medical centers, and research institutions with specialized research interest, and in many cases, clinical expertise in the management of the specific medical condition. The "Centers of Research" directory is a valuable resource for quickly identifying and locating leading medical authorities and medical institutions within the United States and other countries that are considered to be at the forefront in clinical research and treatment of the condition.

Inclusion of the names of specific doctors, researchers, hospitals, medical centers, or research institutions in this *Guidebook* does not imply endorsement by Medifocus.com, Inc. or any of its affiliates. Consumers are encouraged to conduct additional research to identify health-care professionals, hospitals, and medical institutions with expertise in providing specific medical advice, guidance, and treatment for this condition.

Section 5 - Tips on Finding and Choosing a Doctor

One of the most important decisions confronting patients who have been diagnosed with a serious medical condition is finding and choosing a qualified physician who will deliver high-level, quality medical care in accordance with curently accepted guidelines and standards of care. Finding the "best" doctor to manage your condition, however, can be a frustrating and time-consuming experience unless you know what you are looking for and how to go about finding it. This section of your Guidebook offers important tips for how to find physicians as well as suggestions for how to make informed choices about choosing a doctor who is right for you.

Section 6 - Directory of Organizations

This section of your *Guidebook* is a directory of select disease organizations and support groups that are in the business of helping patients and their families by providing access to information, resources, and services. Many of these organizations can answer your questions, enable you to network with other patients, and help you find a doctor in your

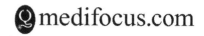

geographical area who specializes in managing your condition.

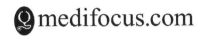
medifocus.com

Ordering Full-Text Articles

After reviewing your *MediFocus Guidebook*, you may wish to order the full-text copy of some of the journal article citations that are referenced in the *Guidebook*. There are several options available for obtaining full-text copies of journal articles, however, with the exception of obtaining the article yourself by visiting a nearby medical library, most involve a fee to cover the costs of photocopying, delivering, and paying the copyright royalty fees set by the individual publishers of medical journals.

This section of your *MediFocus Guidebook* provides some basic information about how you can go about obtaining full-text copies of journal articles from various fee-based document delivery resources.

Commercial Document Delivery Services

There are numerous commercial document delivery companies that provide full-text photocopying and delivery services to the general public. The costs may vary from company to company so it is worth your while to carefully shop-around and compare prices. Some of these commercial document delivery services enable you to order articles directly online from the company's web site. You can locate companies that provide document delivery services by typing the key words "document delivery" into any major Internet search engine.

National Library of Medicine's "Loansome Doc" Document Retrieval Services

The National Library of Medicine (NLM), located in Bethesda, Maryland, offers full-text photocopying and delivery of journal articles through its on-line service known as "Loansome Doc". To learn more about how you can order articles using "Loansome Doc", please visit the NLM web site at:
http://www.nlm.nih.gov/pubs/factsheets/loansome_doc.html

Participating "Loansome Doc" Libraries: United States

In the United States there are approximately 250 medical libraries that participate in the National Library of Medicine's "Loansome Doc" document retrieval and delivery services for the general public. Please note that each participating library sets its own policies and

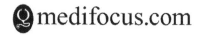

charges for providing document retrieval services. To order full-text copies of articles, simply contact a participating "Loansome Doc" medical library in your geographical area and ask to speak with one of the reference librarians. They can answer all of your questions including fees, delivery options, and turn-around time.

Here is how to find a participating "Loansome Doc" library in the U.S. that provides article retrieval services for the general public:

- **United States** - Contact a Regional Medical Library at 1-800-338-7657 (Monday - Friday; 8:30 AM - 5:30 PM). They will provide information about libraries in your area with which you may establish an account for the "Loansome Doc" service.

- **Canada** - Contact the Canada Institute for Scientific and Technical Information (CISTI) at 1-800-668-1222 for information about libraries in your area.

International MEDLARS Centers

If you reside outside the United States, you can obtain copies of medical journal articles through one of several participating International Medical Literature Analysis and Retrieval Systems (MEDLARS) Centers that provide "Loansome Doc" services in over 20 major countries. International MEDLARS Centers can be found in some of these countries: Australia, Canada, China, Egypt, France, Germany, Hong Kong, India, Israel, Italy, Japan, Korea, Kuwait, Mexico, Norway, Russia, South Africa, Sweden, and the United Kingdom. A complete listing of International MEDLARS Centers, including locations and telephone contact information can be viewed at:
http://www.nlm.nih.gov/pubs/factsheets/intlmedlars.html

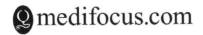 medifocus.com

NOTES

Use this page for taking notes as you review your Guidebook

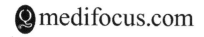

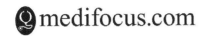

2 - The Intelligent Patient Overview

NON-HODGKIN'S LYMPHOMA

Introduction to Non-Hodgkin's Lymphoma

The Lymphatic System

The *lymphatic system* represents the body's primary defense mechanism against invasion by foreign, potentially disease-producing microorganisms such as bacteria, viruses, and fungi. In humans, the lymphatic system includes the following components:

- Lymph Nodes - These are pea-sized nodules that are found throughout the lymphatic system and are especially abundant in the groin, armpits, abdomen, and neck areas. Lymph nodes serve to filter-out dead microorganisms that are destroyed by the body's immune system.

- Lymphatic Vessels - The lymphatic vessels are a series of channels or conduits similar to veins that carry a colorless liquid called *lymph* that is filtered and collected from the body's organs and tissues. Lymphatic fluid contains a rich supply of specialized white blood cells called *lymphocytes* that are the key cells of the body's immune system.

- Lymphocytes - There are two major types of lymphocytes known as B-lymphoyctes and T-lymphocytes. B-lymphocytes are produced in the bone marrow and regulate or control the production of antibodies - specialized proteins that bind to the surface of microorganisms and facilitate their destruction by other specialized cells of the body's immune system. This type of immunity is called *humoral immunity* or *antibody-mediated immunity* because antibodies that are produced by B-lymphocytes are the key cells involved in fighting off the invading microorganisms. There are five major types of antibodies, also called *immunoglobulins*, produced by B-lymphocytes: IgG, IgM, IgA, IgD, and IgE.

T-lymphocytes are specialized white blood cells that are produced in the bone marrow and mature in the *thymus gland*, a small gland located in the chest just below the sternum (breastbone). T-lymphocytes are responsible for a type of immunity called *cell-mediated immunity*. This type of immunity plays an important role in:

- Destruction of the body's cells that have been infected by bacteria, viruses, or fungi

- Destruction of altered (mutated) cells that arise during the course of normal cell division in the body that can potentially turn into cancer cells

Other Components of the Lymphatic System

Other organs of the body that contain lymphatic tissue include:

- Spleen - The large oval-shaped organ on the left side of the body between the stomach and diaphragm that stores red blood cells and white blood cells that are involved in immune responses.

- Thymus gland - A small gland located in the chest just below the breastbone that is involved in the maturation of T-lymphocytes.

- Bone marrow - The soft innermost portion of bone that produces red and white blood cells.

- Tonsils - These are lymphoid organs located at the back of the throat that help the body defend itself against upper respiratory tract infections.

- Adenoids - These are two groups of lymphoid tissue that lie on either side of and at the very back of the throat. In children, the adenoids are thought to be involved in immune responses to infection but, as a person ages, the adenoids shrink in size until they disappear and are, therefore, not likely to be important in protecting against infection.

Functions of the Lymphatic System

The three primary functions of the lymphatic system include:

- Host Defense and Immunity - protecting the body from invasion by foreign organisms

- Maintaining fluid balance in the body by filtering and collecting fluids and proteins from the lymph and returning it back into the bloodstream.

- Absorbing lipids (fats) from the gut and transporting it to the bloodstream.

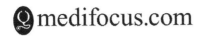 medifocus.com

What is Non-Hodgkin's Lymphoma?

The word "lymphoma" is a general term used to describe a variety of cancers that affect the lymphatic system. Lymphomas originate in the lymphoid tissue of the lymphatic system and are composed of either B or T lymphocytes. Lymphomas tend to form solid tumors in the body and are often felt as a painless lump that can occur almost anywhere in the body.

The two major types of lymphomas include *Hodgkin's disease* (now known as Hodgkin's lymphoma) and *non-Hodgkin's lymphoma* (NHL). In general, these two types of lymphomas can be differentiated by examining the cancer cells under a microscope. The cancer cells in the lymphatic tissues of patients with Hodgkin's disease contain specific cells called *Reed-Sternberg cells* that are not found in patients with non-Hodgkin's lymphoma. Approximately 85% of all non-Hodgkin's lymphomas originate in B-lymphocytes and are sometimes referred to as *B-cell lymphomas*.

Non-Hodgkin's lymphoma represents the most common type of cancers of the blood-forming tissues (hematologic malignancies) and is currently the 6th leading cause of cancer death in the United States. Approximately 60,000 new cases of non-Hodgkin's lymphoma are diagnosed in the U.S. each year with about 95% of these cases occurring in adults 40 to 70 years of age. The disease affects men more frequently than women with about 60% of cases occurring in males and 40% in females. Approximately 25,000 deaths occur each year in the U.S. that are attributed to non-Hodgkin's lymphoma. Epidemiological studies have found that the disease is more common in whites than in African Americans or Asians and clusters of the disease have been found in areas of the U.S. where HIV infection, the virus that causes AIDS, is prevalent.

What Causes Non-Hodgkin's Lymphoma?

Despite the identification of certain risk factors for non-Hodgkin's lymphoma (discussed in detail in the next section), most patients who develop non-Hodgkin's lymphoma (NHL) do not belong to any of these high-risk categories. Although major advances have been made in our understanding of the biology and physiology of cancers in general, currently, researchers still do not completely understand the basic scientific question of what causes a normal lymphocyte to become transformed into a cancerous lymphoma cell. What researchers do know with some degree of certainty is that mutations (alterations) in the DNA - the body's genetic code that regulates cellular function and controls the inheritance of characteristics - can speed up the rate of cell division through specific genes that can turn a normal cell into a cancer cell.

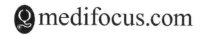

In addition to mutations in the DNA, scientists also believe that non-Hodgkin's lymphoma may be caused by a mechanism called *DNA translocation*. This occurs when DNA from one of the 23 pairs of chromosomes in a normal cell breaks off and "translocates" (moves) by attaching to a different chromosome. This new, abnormal chromosome is thought to trigger the sequence of cellular events that eventually lead to the development of non-Hodgkin's lymphoma.

Risk Factors for Non-Hodgkin's Lymphoma

A variety of risk factors have been identified for the development of non-Hodgkin's lymphoma (NHL), however, as mentioned previously, most patients have no known risk factors. The risk factors for non-Hodgkin's lymphoma can be grouped as follows:

- Autoimmune Disorders - Patients with certain autoimmune disorders, where the body's immune system attacks its own tissues and organs, are at higher risk for developing non-Hodgkin's lymphoma. Examples include:

  - Systemic lupus erythematosus
  - Rheumatoid arthritis
  - Hashimoto's thyroiditis
  - Sjogren's syndrome

- HIV Infection - Patients who are infected with the HIV virus, the virus that is thought to be the cause of AIDS, are at higher risk for developing non-Hodgkin's lymphoma.

- Immunosuppressive Drug Therapy - Patients receiving organ transplants who require treatment with drugs that suppress the immune system are at higher risk for developing non-Hodgkin's lymphoma.

- Infectious Disease Agents - Infection with certain microorganisms is thought to play a role in the development of non-Hodgkin's lymphoma. Examples include:

  - Helicobacter pylori - a bacterium that has been linked to primary gastric (stomach) lymphoma.
  - Epstein-Barr virus - a virus that has been linked to a specific subtype of non-Hodgkin's lymphoma called Burkitt's lymphoma.
  - HTLV-1 - this virus has been implicated in patients with T-cell lymphoma and leukemia.
  - HIV - the virus that is believed to be the cause of AIDS.

- Chemical Exposure - Exposure to certain chemicals is thought to increase the risk for

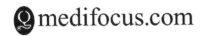

developing non-Hodgkin's lymphoma. Examples include:

- Benzene
- Formaldehyde
- Paint thinners
- Styrene
- Lead
- Herbicides and pesticides

- Older Age - The risk of developing non-Hodgkin's lymphoma increases with age with about 95% of cases occurring in patients between the ages of 40 to 70.

- Male Gender - The risk of developing non-Hodgkin's lymphoma is higher among men than women with a ratio of about 1.4 to 1.0.

- Race - Epidemiological studies have found that non-Hodgkin's lymphoma is more common in whites than in African Americans or Asians.

Classification of Non-Hodgkin's Lymphoma

It should be noted that non-Hodgkin's lymphoma (NHL) is not a single disease but includes a heterogeneous (diverse) group of diseases, each of which carries a different prognosis (outlook). Over the years, several different classification systems have been developed to classify non-Hodgkin's lymphomas including:

- International Working Formulation (IWF) Classification System
- Revised European-American Classification of Lymphoid Neoplasms (REAL)
- Ann Arbor Staging System

International Working Formulation Classification System

The International Working Formulation (IWF) classification system loosely groups non-Hodgkin's lymphomas into the following 3 grades:

- Low-grade lymphomas - these are slow-growing lymphomas that are also referred to as *indolent lymphomas*.

- Intermediate-grade lymphomas - these are considered to be moderately aggressive lymphomas.

- High-grade lymphomas - these lymphomas are considered to be more aggressive

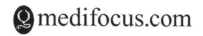

than the intermediate-grade lymphomas.

Revised European-American Classification of Lymphoid Neoplasms

The Revised European-American Classification of Lymphoid Neoplasms (REAL) classification system is based upon the cellular type of the lymphocytes that are affected by the lymphoma. In general, the REAL classification system groups non-Hodgkin's lymphomas as follows:

- B-cell lymphomas - if B-lymphocytes are affected
- T-cell lymphomas - if T-lymphocytes are affected.

Ann Arbor Staging System

"Staging" is a system used by doctors to evaluate the extent of spread of a cancer and is an important factor in determining both the type of treatment as well as predicting the prognosis. Patients with non-Hodgkin's lymphoma are usually staged by the Ann Arbor staging system which evaluates two major factors:

- Site (location) of the lymphoma
- Presence or absence of clinical symptoms.

The Ann Arbor staging system classifies patients with non-Hodgkin's lymphoma into one of the following four stages (categories):

- Stage I - The lymphoma is only present in a single region of the body and involves either a single lymph node region (e.g., groin, neck, armpit) or a single organ outside the lymphatic system (extralymphatic involvement).

- Stage II - The lymphoma affects two or more lymph node regions on the same side of the *diaphragm* (the large muscle attached to the rib cage that is involved in breathing) or the lymphoma has spread from the lymph node into the surrounding tissue.

- Stage III - The lymphoma affects lymph node areas on both sides of the diaphragm and may have also spread to the surrounding tissue or the spleen.

- Stage IV - Patients in this category have lymphoma that affects one or more organs outside of the lymphatic system (extralymphatic lymphoma). Lymphoma cells may or may not be present in nearby lymph nodes. Stage IV disease represents a disseminated (widespread) form of non-Hodgkin's lymphoma.

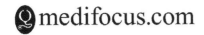

The Ann Arbor classification system also takes into consideration whether symptoms of non-Hodgkin's lymphoma are present or absent. Patients without symptoms are designated with the letter "A" while those with symptoms are designated with the letter "B". The letters "A" or "B" are added to the stage designation (stage I through stage IV) as a means of further classifying the extent of the non-Hodgkin's lymphoma. An international group of lymphoma experts has incorporated the Ann Arbor staging classification along with other clinical attributes to predict overall prognosis and survival (see Prognosis for Non-Hodgkin's Lymphoma section). This staging system is useful for both aggressive and indolent non-Hodgkin's lymphoma.

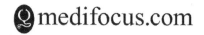medifocus.com

Diagnosis of Non-Hodgkin's Lymphoma

Signs and Symptoms of Non-Hodgkin's Lymphoma

Signs and symptoms of non-Hodgkin's lymphoma (NHL) include:

- Lymphadenopathy - a painless swelling of lymph nodes in any area of the body - is the most common symptom of non-Hodgkin's lymphoma.

    - In most cases, especially in children, swollen lymph nodes are due to an infection and usually disappear once the infection has been eradicated.

    - Patients with non-Hodgkin's lymphoma have enlarged lymph nodes (> 1.0 cm) that persists for at least 6 weeks.

    - Patients with non-Hodgkin's lymphoma of the abdomen usually have a swollen, distended abdomen.

- Enlargement of the liver (hepatomegaly) or enlargement of the spleen (splenomegaly)

- Chest Pain - if the lymphoma affects the lymphoid tissue of the thymus gland (located near the breastbone), the swelling of the thymus gland may cause chest pain.

- General Symptoms - One or more of the following general symptoms may or may not be present in patients with non-Hodgkin's lymphoma:

    - shortness of breath
    - generalized feeling of weakness or fatigue
    - profuse sweating (particularly while sleeping at night)
    - loss of appetite or unexplained weight loss
    - severe itching
    - recurrent infections
    - easily bruised skin

Diagnostic Testing for Non-Hodgkin's Lymphoma

Medical History and Physical Examination

- The physician will take a thorough medical history to uncover any signs/symptoms of non-Hodgkin's lymphoma as well as determine any possible risk factors for the disease.

- A complete physical examination of the patient is then performed by the physician who will pay particular attention to the presence of swollen lymph nodes and possible enlargement of the liver and/or spleen.

Laboratory Evaluation

Your physician will also take a sample of your blood and submit it to the laboratory for further studies including:

- Complete blood count (CBC)
- Comprehensive metabolic panel to monitor electrolytes and assess kidney and liver function
- Measurement of levels of specific blood components (LDH, uric acid, and beta-2 microglobulin) to determine the tumor burden (the amount of cancer cells that are present in the body).
- HIV testing is standard of care in working-up patients with non-Hodgkin's lymphoma and Hodgkin's lymphoma. Using standard chemotherapy regimens on individuals who are HIV-positive can lead to serious complications or death. Your physician is not necessarily ordering an HIV test because he/she believes that you have AIDS but is rather trying to provide optimal care and treatment.

Imaging Studies

- Chest X-ray
- Computed tomography (CT) of the chest, abdomen, and pelvis
- In some cases, specialized imaging studies such as a *gallium scan* or, more often, *positron emission tomography* (PET) imaging may be recommended for the staging of non-Hodgkin's lymphoma or Hodgkin's lymphoma.

Lymph Node Biopsy

In cases where an enlarged lymph node persists for 6-weeks or longer and the physician suspects lymphoma, a lymph node biopsy will be required and the tissue will be submitted to a pathology laboratory to determine the presence or absence of lymphoma cells. Lymph node biopsy is the only definitive way to diagnose non-Hodgkin's lymphoma and several different biopsy procedures are available. Before undergoing a lymph node biopsy, you will want to discuss with your surgeon in detail the various biopsy options including the advantages and disadvantages of each technique as well as the potential risks and complications. In general, the biopsy techniques available for the diagnosis of non-Hodgkin's lymphoma include:

- Surgical Biopsy - either the entire lymph node or a piece of the lymph node is removed surgically. The biopsy specimen is then submitted to the pathology laboratory and examined under a microscope to look for the presence of lymphoma cells.

- Fine Needle Aspiration (FNA) Biopsy - a very thin needle (biopsy needle) is inserted into the area of the tumor and tissue is withdrawn into a syringe. The biopsy specimen is then submitted to the pathology laboratory and examined under a microscope to look for the presence of lymphoma cells.

- Large Needle/Core Biopsy - This technique uses a large-bore needle to obtain a sample of tissue but is not widely used for the diagnosis of non-Hodgkin's lymphoma. It is usually reserved for patients who cannot tolerate a surgical biopsy.

- Other Biopsy Procedures - Once lymphoma has been diagnosed, your physician may recommend additional biopsy procedures to help determine the stage or the extent of spread of the disease. These may include a *bone marrow biopsy* to determine if the lymphoma has spread to the bone marrow, and a *lumbar puncture* (spinal tap) to determine if the lymphoma has affected the central nervous system (brain and spinal cord).

Special Laboratory Tests

Tissue samples removed at the time of biopsy from patients with non-Hodgkin's lymphoma will be also subjected to several special tests in the pathology laboratory to help doctors identify the type of non-Hodgkin's lymphoma that is causing the disease. These tests include:

- Immunophenotyping - This special immunological test uses antibodies to detect and identify specific markers called "antigens" that may be present on the surface of lymphoma cells. If certain surface antigens are identified, the oncologist may choose to use monoclonal antibodies such as rituximab (Rituxan) to treat the lymphoma.

- Cytogenetics - Lymphoma cells are examined under a microscope to look for abnormalities in the chromosomes such as DNA translocations or extra pairs of chromosomes.

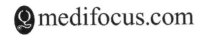

Treatment Options for Non-Hodgkin's Lymphoma

The treatment options for patients with non-Hodgkin's lymphoma (NHL) depend upon a variety of factors including the grade of the lymphoma (low, intermediate, or high), the stage of the disease, the site of involvement, as well as the age and general health of the patient. All of these facts are taken into consideration in developing an individualized treatment plan for the patient with non-Hodgkin's lymphoma.

The treatment of non-Hodgkin's lymphoma requires a multidisciplinary approach, meaning that several doctors from various medical specialties are involved in the management of the patient. These usually include a hematologist/oncologist (cancer specialist), radiation oncologist (a doctor who specializes in administering radiation therapy for cancer), an oncology nurse (a nurse who administers chemotherapy and monitors the patient during chemotherapy sessions), a social worker, and a mental health professional who can help the patient better cope with the psychological and emotional aspects of battling lymphoma. Ideally, all of these medical specialists should work closely with your primary care physician to keep him/her apprised of your treatment and progress.

Treatment Options for Low-Grade Non-Hodgkin's Lymphomas

Watchful Waiting

Because low-grade lymphomas are indolent and grow slowly, a standard option recommended to newly diagnosed patients with low tumor burden and no symptoms is "watchful waiting". This approach is also referred to as "deferred initial therapy" because initial treatment is deferred (delayed) until the lymphoma progresses and/or the patient develops symptoms of lymphoma. It is important to note that even newly diagnosed patients with low-grade lymphoma who elect the "watchful waiting" option will eventually require treatment for their disease. The critical decision that has to be made during the "watchful waiting" period is when to initiate treatment. During this period, patients have to be monitored closely for progression of the disease and signs/symptoms of non-Hodgkin's lymphoma and, once these develop, primary therapy is started.

Chemotherapy

Numerous chemotherapeutic drugs are available for the treatment of non-Hodgkin's lymphomas. Depending upon the type and stage of lymphoma, chemotherapy may involve the use of a single drug (monotherapy) or a combination of drugs (combination chemotherapy). Patients with low-grade lymphoma with early stage disease (Stage I or II) are usually treated with single agent chemotherapy (e.g., chlorambucil, fludarabine, or rituximab). Patients with more advanced disease (Stage III or IV) usually require combination chemotherapy with several anticancer drugs that are given during the same treatment session. Examples of drug combinations that are commonly used to treat non-Hodgkin's lymphoma include:

- CHOP: cyclophosphamide/doxorubicin/vincristine/prednisone
- CVP: cyclophosphamide/vincristine/prednisone

In general, chemotherapy is administered on an outpatient basis in 3 to 6 cycles that are given at 21 to 28 day intervals. Common side-effects of chemotherapy, that are usually temporary and resolve once chemotherapy has been completed, may include:

- Alopecia (hair loss)
- Mucositis (mouth sores caused by inflammation of the mucous membranes lining of the mouth)
- Nausea and/or vomiting
- Increased susceptibility to infection due to decreased numbers of white blood cells that are affected by the chemotherapy
- Increased susceptibility to bruising and bleeding due to decreased numbers of platelets (blood cells involved in blood clotting) that are affected by the chemotherapy
- Loss of appetite
- Generalized feeling of fatigue
- Peripheral neuropathy - a disorder of the peripheral nerves characterized by symptoms of numbness, tingling or burning sensations, pain, and weakness. These symptoms can affect the feet, hands, legs, arms, or face. This condition is caused by the vincristine component of the CHOP chemotherapy regimen.

Radiation Therapy

External beam radiation therapy is a treatment that uses high-energy x-rays from a radioactive source to destroy cancer cells. The radiation beams from outside the patient's body are targeted to the area of the body that is affected by the cancer. Radiation therapy for non-Hodgkin's lymphoma is usually administered once or twice a day for 5 to 8 weeks depending upon the total dosage that is required.

For patients with low-grade lymphoma with early stage disease (Stage I or II), radiation therapy may be the primary method of treatment. It has been estimated that radiation therapy is curative in about 50% of these patients. In many cases, radiation therapy is combined with chemotherapy. Common, usually temporary, side-effects of radiation therapy may include:

- Generalized fatigue
- Red, dry, tender, or itchy skin near the area of irradiation
- Dry/sore throat and difficulty swallowing if the chest or neck area is the site of irradiation
- Nausea, vomiting, or diarrhea in cases of radiation therapy to the abdomen
- Increased susceptibility to infection due to decreased numbers of white blood cells that are affected by the radiation therapy.

Treatment Options for Intermediate-Grade and High-Grade Non-Hodgkin's Lymphomas

The treatment options for intermediate-grade and high-grade lymphomas, which tend to be more aggressive, are much more straightforward than those for the low-grade (indolent) lymphomas. Combination chemotherapy with CHOP (cyclophosphamide/doxorubicin/vincristine/prednisone) is considered as standard treatment for intermediate-grade and high-grade lymphomas.

For patients with early stage disease (Stage I or II), CHOP chemotherapy is usually followed by localized external-beam radiation therapy. Although CHOP is the standard regimen, your cancer specialist may elect to use a different combination of anticancer drugs in place of CHOP especially if your type of lymphoma is considered to be very aggressive. Examples of these chemotherapeutic regimens include:

- m-BACOD - bleomycin/doxorubicin/cyclosphosphamide/vincristine/dexamethasone/ methotrexate/leucovorin
- ProMACE - prednisone/methotrexate/leucovorin/doxorubicin/cyclophosphamide /etoposide
- CytaBOM-cytarabine/bleomycin/vincristine/methotrexate

Despite the availability of these newer chemotherapeutic regimens, research has shown no benefits in terms of either efficacy (cure rate) or survival between these newer agents and CHOP. However, because these newer regimens are more toxic (cause more side-effects) and are more costly, CHOP remains the standard regimen of choice in most cases. CHOP is also considered the standard chemotherapeutic regimen for patients with intermediate-grade or high-grade lymphomas with more advanced disease (Stage III or IV). In patients over the age of 60, CHOP chemotherapy may be combined with immunotherapy using a monoclonal antibody such as rituximab (Rituxan).

Currently, the standard of care for the treatment of intermediate-grade (diffuse large B cell) lymphoma is rituximab combined with CHOP or a similar regimen such as those listed above. Patients receiving rituximab as part of their regimen have higher survival and

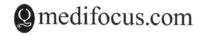

remission rates than those not receiving rituximab. Also, some physicians now administer CHOP chemotherapy every 2-weeks instead of the usual (standard) every 3-weeks dosing schedule. This is termed "dose defense" chemotherapy and may be more effective for elderly patients with intermediate-grade non-Hodgkin's lymphoma. A myeloid growth factor called *pegfilgrastim* (Neulasta) must be given when using the shorter 14-day chemotherapy cycle. Otherwise, the white blood cells would not recover sufficiently between chemotherapy cycles to enable the use of the shorter-interval dosing schedule.

New Treatments for Non-Hodgkin's Lymphoma

Although some improvement in the treatment of non-Hodgkin's lymphoma (NHL) has been made in recent years, it has become increasingly clear that the currently available chemotherapeutic regimens are not curative for many patients, especially those with advanced (disseminated) disease. This has led to the search for newer treatment approaches in an effort to increase survival rates. Some of the newer treatments for non-Hodgkin's lymphomas that are currently being investigated include:

- Immunotherapy (Biological Therapy)
- Proteosome Inhibitors
- Purine Analogues

Immunotherapy

- Interferon-alpha - Interferons are a group of proteins produced by cells that have been infected by a virus that help the body mount an effective immune response in order to eliminate the infecting virus. Interferons can also reduce the growth and multiplication of cancer cells. One type of interferon that is being investigated as immunotherapy for certain types of non-Hodgkin's lymphomas is interferon-alpha. Although some studies have shown that interferon-alpha can cause some types of non-Hodgkin's lymphoma tumors to shrink, its role in the treatment of non-Hodgkin's lymphoma is still considered experimental.

- Monoclonal Antibody Therapy - Monoclonal antibodies are specialized proteins produced in the laboratory that are designed to specifically attach to and, with the help of the immune system, destroy lymphoma cells. One example of a monoclonal antibody that is being used for the treatment of non-Hodgkin's lymphoma is rituximab (Rituxan). Rituximab is a monoclonal antibody that preferentially seeks out and binds (attaches) to certain types of lymphoma cells that express (produce) a specific surface antigen called the CD 20 antigen. Rituximab has been approved by the U.S. Food and Drug Administration (FDA) for the treatment of relapsed or refractory B-cell lymphomas that express the CD 20 surface antigen. Another monoclonal antibody called Campath is being used for patients with the more

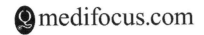

uncommon T-cell type non-Hodgkin's lymphoma. Campath is usually combined with other therapy such as CHOP or a nucleoside analogue such as pentostatin.

In June and July 2004, Biogen Idec and Genentech notified healthcare professionals of revisions to the WARNINGS section of the prescribing information for rituximab (Rituxan) due to reports of Hepatitis B virus (HBV) reactivation with fulminant hepatitis, hepatic failure, and death in some patients with hematologic malignancies. Persons at high risk of HBV infection should be screened before initiation of Rituxan. Carriers of hepatitis B should be closely monitored for clinical and laboratory signs of active HBV infection and for signs of hepatitis during and for up to several months following Rituxan therapy.

Despite this warning, several investigators believe that the benefit of rituximab is so significant that they are placing patients who are HBV antigen-positive on anti-viral therapy before starting treatment with rituximab. Certainly, your doctor should have a frank discussion with you weighing the risks and benefits of such an approach if you are found to be HBV antigen-positive and rituximab is being considered in the treatment protocol.

- Radioimmunotherapy - This is a specific type of immunotherapy with a monoclonal antibody that is "conjugated" (bound to) a radioactive compound known as an *isotope*. When administered to a patient with non-Hodgkin's lymphoma, the monoclonal antibody preferentially binds to lymphoma cells and the conjugated radioactive substance that is bound to the antibody destroys the lymphoma cells. Examples of conjugated monoclonal antibodies that are being investigated for the treatment of certain types of non-Hodgkin's lymphomas include:

    - ibritumomab tiuxetan (Zevalin) - a monoclonal antibody that is conjugated with radioactive yttrium (YT-90).
    - tositumomab (Bexxar) - a monoclonal antibody that is conjugated with radioactive iodine (I-131).

Proteosome Inhibitors

A new class of drugs called *proteosome inhibitors* has been approved for treatment of a lymphoid malignancy called *multiple myeloma*. A drug belonging to the class of proteosome inhibitors called Velcade has been very effective for controlling multiple myeloma even in patients who had received intensive chemotherapy and were thought to be resistant to further chemotherapy. Velcade is now being evaluated in several types of non-Hodgkin's lymphoma and is expected to be incorporated into many of the non-Hodgkin's lymphoma chemotherapy regimens in the near future.

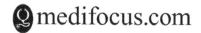

Purine Analogues

Although purine analogues were developed in the early 1950's as a novel class of anticancer drugs, they have recently received significant attention for the targeted treatment of certain types of non-Hodgkin's lymphomas. These drugs work by preventing cells from producing *purine* - a compound that is an integral component of DNA. Examples of purine analogues include:

- Fludarabine
- Cladribine
- Pentostatin

Salvage Chemotherapy for Non-Hodgkin's Lymphoma

Salvage chemotherapy is chemotherapy that is given after recurrence of a tumor (relapsed disease). Both salvage and/or high-dose chemotherapy are usually considered as a treatment option for patients with aggressive non-Hodgkin's lymphoma (NHL) who either fail to respond to standard treatment (refractory disease) or whose lymphoma recurs either during or after completion of standard therapy (relapsed disease). Salvage chemotherapy involves the use of combinations of high-doses of anticancer drugs which may include:

- ESHAP: methylprednisolone, etoposide, cytarabine, cisplatin
- DHAP: cisplatin, cytarabine, dexamethasone
- EPOCH: etoposide, prednisone, vincristine, cyclophosphamide, doxorubicin
- MIME: mesna, ifosfamide, mitoxantrone, etoposide

Although salvage chemotherapy is a treatment approach that enables doctors to try to eradicate the lymphoma cells with very high doses of anticancer drugs, the lymphoma will usually recur and may be more resistant to chemotherapy. Therefore, a common approach is to use salvage chemotherapy to reduce the amount of disease and then give "consolidation" therapy using very high doses of chemotherapy and/or total body irradiation (TBI). Unfortunately, one of the side-effects of this treatment strategy is that the combination of high doses of potent drugs also destroys the stem cells (blood-forming cells) in the bone marrow that produce red blood cells, white blood cells, and platelets. This can lead to serious, life-threatening complications such as anemia, recurrent infections, and bleeding problems. To overcome this problem, patients with non-Hodgkin's lymphoma who require high-dose chemotherapy may be considered candidates for stem cell transplantation.

Stem Cell Transplantation in Non-Hodgkin's

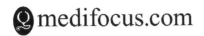
Lymphoma

What are Stem Cells?

Stem cells are immature, special cells located in the *bone marrow* (the spongy material found inside long-bones) that mature into the three major types of blood cells:

- Red blood cells - carry oxygen to all tissues and organs of the body
- White blood cells - components of the body's immune system responsible for fighting infections
- Platelets - specialized cells in the bloodstream that are responsible for clotting of blood (stop bleeding when a person sustains a cut or an injury to blood vessels)

High-dose chemotherapy used to destroy cancer cells, unfortunately, also kills most the patient's blood-forming bone marrow and stem cells. Without these critical cells, the patient is susceptible to a variety of potentially life-threatening problems including increased susceptibility to infections and bleeding complications. Bone marrow and stem cell transplantation enables doctors to replace the critical blood-forming cells after high-dose chemotherapy to kill cancer cells has been completed.

The source of stem cells used for transplantation is either bone marrow usually harvested (removed) from the hip bone (*bone marrow transplantation*) or the stem cells can be obtained from the peripheral bloodstream via a procedure called *apheresis* (*peripheral blood stem cell transplantation*). In both cases, the stem cells are frozen and stored for later use until the patient has completed their course of high-dose chemotherapy and are then administered to the patient by intravenous infusion. For the purposes of this discussion the terms "bone marrow transplantation" and "stem cell transplantation" are used interchangeably.

Many times, salvage regimens such as DHAP and MIME can generate sufficient stem cells to be harvested and saved for high-dose chemotherapy procedures. Other times, large doses of cyclophosphamide and myeloid growth factors, alone or in combination, generate sufficient stem cells in the bloodstream for harvesting and use after high-dose chemotherapy.

There are two primary types of stem cell transplantation procedures:

- Autologous stem cell transplantation
- Allogeneic stem cell transplantation

Autologous Stem Cell Transplantation

In this procedure, the source of the stem cells used for transplantation is the patient who

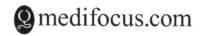

serves as both the "donor" as well as the "recipient". Stem cells are harvested (removed) from the patient's bone marrow or bloodstream before treatment is initiated and the cells are frozen and stored for use after treatment has been completed. A marker on the stem cells called "CD34" can be measured and is a good indicator of having sufficient stem cells for engraftment after high-dose chemotherapy. The patient then undergoes a course of high-dose chemotherapy that is intended to kill the remaining lymphoma cells but also destroys the blood-forming cells in the bone marrow. After the patient completes their course of chemotherapy, the frozen stem cells are thawed and then infused (returned) back into the patient's body by an intravenous infusion.

Allogeneic Stem Cell Transplantation

In this procedure, the source of the stem cells used for transplantation is another person who serves as the "donor". In order to prevent complications related to rejection of the transplanted stem cells, a suitable donor must be identified whose tissue type closely matches that of the recipient. To ensure maximum success of an allogeneic transplant, the donor and recipient's tissue type must be compatible with respect to certain cell antigens or "markers" know as histocompatibility antigens (HLAs). Currently, recipient-donor compatibility for allogeneic stem cell transplantation is determined by a blood test that measures the compatibility or "match" of six different major HLA markers. The most successful allogeneic transplants are achieved in those cases where there is a "perfect match" between the donor and recipient for all six HLA markers. Successful transplants can also be achieved where only 4 or 5 HLA markers match exactly, however, the risk of complications, such as graft-versus-host-disease, is much higher. Close relatives of the patient (such as a brother or sister) are more likely to be an exact or close match than unrelated donors for allogeneic stem cell transplantation. In the event that the patient who requires a stem cell transplant has an identical twin, the twin is an ideal donor because the donor and recipient HLA markers match exactly. This type of stem cell transplant is called a *syngeneic transplant.*

Once a suitable donor has been identified, stem cells are harvested (collected) from either the bone marrow or from the bloodstream and the cells are frozen for later use. Allogeneic bone marrow or peripheral blood stem cells are usually employed "fresh" although they can be frozen, especially if they must be shipped long distances. The patient (transplant recipient) then begins and completes a cycle of high-dose chemotherapy to destroy the remaining lymphoma cells. Patients are also given antirejection drugs such as tacrolimus or cyclosporine (sometimes in combination with prednisone or methotrexate) in order to reduce the likelihood that the patient will reject the donor's transplanted stem cells. The donor's frozen stem cells are then thawed and infused into the recipient via an intravenous line.

Mini-Transplants

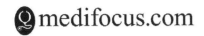

More recently, doctors have developed a newer type of allogeneic stem cell transplantation procedure called mini-transplants. These are also sometimes referred to as *non-myeloablative transplants* or *reduced-intensity transplants*. In contrast to a standard allogeneic stem cell transplant where the goal of treatment is to use high-dose chemotherapy to eradicate the remaining cancer cells and then restore the patient's stem cells that have been also destroyed by the chemotherapy, a mini-transplant uses significantly lower doses of chemotherapy (or radiation) and is, therefore, less toxic to the patient. This lower-dose or reduced-intensity approach kills only some of the remaining cancer cells but does not completely destroy the patient's diseased bone marrow blood-forming cells. The patient then receives a transplant of the donor's bone marrow or stem cells. The donor's transplanted immune cells serve as a "booster" to the recipient's own immune system by recognizing and destroying the remaining cancer cells that have not been killed by the low-dose chemotherapy or radiation therapy. This phenomenon is known as "graft-versus-tumor" effect because the donor's transplanted immune cells are used as a means of targeting and destroying the patient's residual cancer cells.

Although mini-transplants are becoming more common and have been used for patients with a wide range of cancers, they appear to be most effective for patients with *chronic myelogenous leukemia* (CML). The outcome for patients with other types of leukemias, non-Hodgkin's lymphomas, Hodgkin's disease, or multiple myeloma have varied depending upon the type of mini-transplant procedure used. In general, mini-transplants are reserved for older patients (over age 60) or patients with serious underlying conditions who cannot tolerate a standard allogeneic stem cell transplant.

Graft-Versus-Host-Disease

Graft-versus-host-disease (GVHD) is perhaps the most serious potential complication that may develop in patients receiving an allogeneic stem cell transplant. As mentioned previously, in an allogeneic transplant, the source of the stem cells used for transplantation is another individual who serves as the donor. Graft-versus-host disease (GVHD) occurs when the donor's transplanted cells (the graft) begins to attack the recipient's (the host's) own tissues and organs. It should be noted that GVHD can occur with an allogeneic transplant even in cases where the donor and recipient's HLA markers are a "perfect match". This is because currently the degree of compatibility (match) between the donor and recipient is determined on the basis of evaluating similarities of tissue types for six major HLA markers. However, there are other antigens present on the donor's transplanted cells which may differ slightly from those of the recipient's own cells that can lead to the development of GVHD.

GVHD can develop within the first 3 months following allogeneic stem cell transplantation (acute GVHD) or it may develop after 3 months (chronic GVHD). Symptoms of acute GVHD include:

- Itchy, red rash on the hands and feet
- Nausea, diarrhea, and severe stomach cramps
- Jaundice (due to liver damage)

The chronic form of GVHD can be very severe and disabling and, in some cases, may even be fatal. Patients who develop GVHD are treated with various combinations of immunosuppressive drugs such as cyclosporine, methotrexate, and corticosteroids.

In addition to GVHD, other potential complications of bone marrow transplantation include recurrent infections, interstitial pneumonitis, graft failure or rejection, veno-occlusive disease (complete blockage of the central veins of the liver leading to liver damage), and recurrence of the cancer following transplantation.

Prognosis for Non-Hodgkin's Lymphoma

In 1993, a collaborative group known as The International Non-Hodgkin's Lymphoma Prognostic Factors Project published an important article in *The New England Journal of Medicine* (Vol. 329; pp. 987-994) entitled "A Predictive Model for Aggressive Non-Hodgkin's Lymphoma". Based on a study of more than 3,000 patients with diffuse large B-cell lymphoma, these researchers developed an index called the International Prognostic Index (IPI) that is useful in determining the prognosis (outlook) for patients with non-Hodgkin's lymphoma (NHL). Since that time, the IPI has been validated by other studies as being an important prognostic indicator for patients with non-Hodgkin's lymphomas.

The International Prognostic Index (IPI) takes into consideration five major factors or variables that, taken as a whole, can be used by doctors to predict the likely outlook for patients with non-Hodgkin's lymphoma. The five major prognostic factors that are evaluated in the IPI include:

- Age of the Patient - In general, younger patients (age 60 or below) have a better prognosis than older patients over the age of 60.

- Lymphoma Stage - The stage of the lymphoma is an important prognostic indicator because it reflects the extent of spread of the disease. In general, patients with Stage I or II (localized) lymphoma, usually have a more favorable prognosis than those with Stage III or IV (advanced) disease.

- Involvement of Extranodal Sites - This is an indication of whether the lymphoma has affected areas of the body outside of the lymph nodes (extranodal sites). Extranodal sites that may be affected include the bone marrow, lung, liver, spleen, and central nervous system. In general, non-Hodgkin's lymphoma patients with no extranodal site involvement have a better outlook than those patients where the lymphoma has affected one or more extranodal sites.

- Lactate Dehydrogenase Serum Levels - Lactate dehydrogenase (LDH) is an enzyme that can be measured in the blood (serum) that, if elevated above normal levels, can indicate the presence of an aggressive, fast-growing lymphoma. In general, patients with non-Hodgkin's lymphoma with normal levels of LDH usually have a more favorable prognosis than those with elevated LDH serum levels.

- Patient's Performance Status - The term "performance status" refers to the extent of the patient's ability to perform activities of daily living. In other words, the performance status is an indication of the extent to which the disease has affected the patient's lifestyle. Performance status is ranked on a scale from 0 to 4 with a score of "0" or "1" assigned to patients who have good performance status and are capable of maintaining a relatively active lifestyle. In general, non-Hodgkin's lymphoma patients with good performance status have a more favorable prognosis than those with poor performance status.

After evaluating each of the five individual prognostic factors that comprise the IPI, the doctor assigns a score of "1" for each poor prognostic factor. The total IPI score is then determined by adding together all of the poor prognostic factors with a score of "1". The patient is then assigned to one of the following four risk categories:

- Low Risk Category: IPI Score = 0 to 1
- Low/Intermediate Risk Category: IPI Score = 2
- Intermediate/High Risk Category: IPI Score = 3
- High Risk Category : IPI Score = 4 or higher

In general, patients with indolent lymphomas have a relatively good prognosis with a median survival rate of about 10 years. For patients with intermediate-grade to high-grade lymphomas, the 5-year survival rate varies depending upon the IPI risk category. For example, the 5-year survival rate for patients in the low-risk category (IPI Score = 0 to 1) is about 75%, whereas, the 5-year survival rate for patients in the highest risk category (IPI Score = 4 or higher) is about 25%. The overall 5-year survival rate for all IPI risk factor groups combined is about 50%.

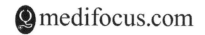medifocus.com

The Role of Complementary and Alternative Therapies in Cancer

Complementary and Alternative Medicine: Definition of Terms

The National Center for Complementary and Alternative Medicine (NCCAM) defines complementary and alternative medicine as "a group of diverse medical and health care systems, practices, and products that are not presently considered to be a part of conventional medicine". The term **complementary medicine** refers to the use of CAM therapies in addition to or in conjunction with conventional mainstream treatments in an "integrative" approach to treatment. The term **alternative medicine**, on the other hand, refers to the use of CAM therapies as a substitute for or in place of conventional mainstream treatments.

Although the terms "complementary" and "alternative" are often used interchangeably by many people when referring to CAM therapies, health care professionals usually make a clear distinction between these two terms. In general, conventional physicians will keep an open mind and tend to support the use of "complementary" therapies in conjunction with standard mainstream treatments while they may resist suggestions for using "alternative" therapies as a substitute for conventional treatments. In fact, many cancer centers in the United States have incorporated select complementary therapies along with standard cancer treatments (e.g., chemotherapy, radiation therapy, surgery) in an emerging field of cancer care known as *integrative oncology*. It is important for patients and their families to keep in mind the very important distinction between the terms "complementary" and "alternative" when discussing the issue of CAM therapies with their health care provider in order to avoid confusion and misunderstandings and ensure effective patient-doctor communication.

The definition of CAM adapted by the NCCAM, which basically defines CAM as any treatment modality, philosophy, or product that falls outside the realm of conventional or standard medical care is well-suited for most Western countries where conventional, modern medicine is the prevailing or predominant health system adapted by the people who live in that culture. For example, conventional or standard treatments for cancer in most modern Western countries include chemotherapy, radiation therapy, biological therapy, and surgery. Other treatment modalities such as acupuncture, hypnotherapy, or the use of shark cartilage would be considered as being outside the realm of conventional medicine and falling under the general umbrella of CAM. The definition of CAM adapted by the NCCAM, however, is more problematic in countries or cultures where a particular

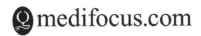

form of CAM, such as Traditional Chinese medicine in China or Ayurvedic medicine in India, represent major health care systems that are recognized, accepted, and utilized by the general population of those countries or cultures.

Care Versus Cure

In discussing the role of CAM therapies for the management of cancer, it is important to differentiate between CAM therapies that purport to "cure" cancer as opposed to those therapies that are used in palliative cancer care to provide relief from cancer-related symptoms and improve the patient's quality of life. Unlike some conventional cancer treatments that have been demonstrated to cure patients with certain types of cancers, currently there is a lack of sufficient scientific evidence to support the conclusion that any specific type of CAM modality can cure cancer. Patients who fail to draw a distinction between the "care versus cure" aspects of CAM therapies may delay seeking or may completely abandon potentially curative mainstream cancer treatments in hope that a particular CAM therapy may be a "magic bullet" for curing their cancer. On the other hand, complementary therapies have become an important aspect of palliative cancer care by helping cancer patients better cope with cancer-related symptoms and side-effects and, thereby, improving quality of life. In fact, many cancer centers in the United States and other Western countries have integrated complementary therapies into their mainstream treatment strategies for palliative cancer care in an emerging field of cancer practice known as *integrative oncology*.

Complementary Therapies for Cancer-Related Symptoms

Conventional cancer treatments such as chemotherapy, radiation therapy, and surgery are often associated with severe side-effects that can significantly impact the patient's quality of life and interfere with routine activities of daily living. In general, side-effects of conventional cancer treatments may include nausea/vomiting, fatigue, anxiety, depression, pain, sleep disturbances, loss of appetite, dry mouth, gastrointestinal disturbances, and peripheral neuropathy. Conventional treatments may not always be completely effective in relieving cancer-related symptoms and, in some cases, the treatments themselves may cause additional side-effects. Complementary therapies, when used in conjunction with conventional mainstream treatments can help patients better cope with cancer-related symptoms and side-effects and also improve physical and emotional well-being and overall quality of life.

Psychological Stress

The diagnosis of cancer is a life-altering event that may evoke feelings of anxiety, fear,

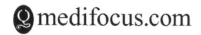

depression, hopelessness, and severe psychological stress in many patients. Studies have shown that about 25% of cancer patients suffer from depression. Conventional treatments for anxiety, stress, and depression may involve the administration of anti-anxiety medications or antidepressants which may cause undesirable side-effects in some patients. Studies have shown that a variety of CAM therapies are useful for controlling anxiety and other mood disturbances when used in conjunction with conventional treatments. These include:

- Mind-body interventions - relaxation techniques, guided-imagery, meditation, hypnosis
- Acupuncture
- Massage therapy
- Music therapy

In general, patients with severe mood disturbances (e.g., panic attacks; suicide ideation) require immediate psychological evaluation and treatment to stabilize their acute condition before CAM therapies may be considered. For most patients with mild to moderate anxiety and mood disturbances, CAM therapies are a useful adjunct to conventional treatments for managing psychological distress. Techniques such as mind-body interventions, acupuncture, and music therapy are generally safe when performed by qualified, experienced practitioners and can help cancer patients better cope with feelings of anxiety, fear, hopelessness, and depression. Although some herbs and dietary supplements (e.g., Kava Kava; St. John's Wort; Passionflower) have been reported to relieve anxiety and mood disturbances, some experts have discouraged the use of these products in cancer patients because they may interfere with drugs used to treat cancer (chemotherapeutic agents) and/or other medications that patients may be taking. Patients should discuss the risks and benefits of using any herbal medications/dietary supplements with their oncologist before taking any of these products, particularly if they are undergoing chemotherapy, radiation therapy, or surgery.

Cancer-Related Pain

Pain is a common symptom that can affect many cancer patients. Most often, the source of the pain is the tumor itself. Cancer-related pain may be caused by spread of the tumor to other tissues and organs or may result from compression of the tumor on a nerve or the spinal cord. In general, *acute* cancer-related pain is most responsive to conventional mainstream treatments which may involve medications (e.g., narcotic analgesics; steroids) or, in severe cases, (e.g., tumor causing spinal cord compression; tumor associated with abdominal obstruction), emergent surgery may be required to relieve the acute pain.

As a general rule, CAM therapies are usually not considered as a viable treatment option for the management of acute cancer-related pain. Once the acute pain has been brought under control by conventional treatment modalities, CAM therapies may be considered in

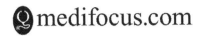

the management of *chronic* cancer-related pain. A potential benefit of using CAM therapies in conjunction with conventional treatments for the management of chronic cancer-related pain is that they may reduce the dosage of conventional pain medications that may be required to achieve chronic pain control and, therefore, also potentially reduce the side-effects that may be associated with conventional pain medications.

A variety of CAM therapies, when used in conjunction with conventional treatments, may be beneficial for the management of cancer-related pain, including:

- Meditation
- Guided imagery
- Hypnosis
- Relaxation techniques
- Massage therapy
- Reflexology
- Acupuncture
- Yoga
- Aromatherapy

Some procedures that may be used for the diagnosis and treatment of some types of cancers may also be associated with pain. Examples include:

- Biopsy - a piece of tissue is removed from the tumor and is examined under a microscope to determine if it is malignant or benign.
- Placement of a central line catheter that is used to administer chemotherapeutic agents and/or other medications
- Bone marrow aspiration
- Lumbar puncture

A variety of CAM therapies, particularly mind-body techniques, have been found to be beneficial for controlling pain associated with cancer-related procedures (both diagnostic and therapeutic), especially in children with cancer, although they appear to be useful in adults as well.

Some cancer patients who undergo surgery to remove a tumor develop persistent neuropathic pain due to injury of nerves during the surgical procedure. In general, severe neuropathic pain may be difficult to control with conventional pain management treatment modalities. There is some evidence that acupuncture, when used in conjunction with conventional pain management strategies, may be effective for the management of persistent neuropathic pain that may develop in some patients after cancer surgery.

Nausea and Vomiting

Nausea and vomiting are relatively common side-effects in patients undergoing cancer chemotherapy. When used in conjunction with standard treatments, CAM therapies may offer patients additional relief from chemotherapy-induced nausea and vomiting. A 1998 National Institutes of Health (NIH) Consensus Conference concluded that there is clear evidence supporting the efficacy of acupuncture for controlling nausea and vomiting associated with cancer chemotherapy. Other CAM therapies that may help cancer patients better cope with chemotherapy-induced nausea and vomiting include:

- Acupressure
- Aromatherapy
- Hypnosis
- Guided imagery
- Music therapy
- Massage therapy

Other Cancer-Related Symptoms

There is a limited amount of evidence which suggests that CAM therapies may be useful for helping patients to better cope with a variety of other common cancer-related symptoms including:

- Fatigue - A study published in 2004 in the *Journal of Clinical Oncology* (Vol. 22, Issue 9; pp. 1731-1735) reported that acupuncture reduced chemotherapy-related fatigue by 31% after 6 weeks of acupuncture treatment.

- Dry Mouth (*xerostomia*) - Several studies suggest that acupuncture may be useful in the management of dry mouth that occurs in some patients undergoing radiation therapy to the head and neck.

- Hot Flashes - Some women with breast cancer who are treated with a drug called *tamoxifen* may experience hot flashes that can be very uncomfortable. A study published in 2002 in the journal *Tumori* (Volume 88, Issue 2; pp. 128-130) reported that acupuncture may relieve menopause-related symptoms, including hot flashes, in women taking tamoxifen.

- Lymphedema - A study published in 2002 in the *European Journal of Cancer Care* (Volume 11; Issue 4, pp. 254-261) reported that a specific type of massage therapy known as *manual lymphatic drainage* (MLD) was beneficial for the treatment of breast cancer related lymphedema and also improved overall quality of life.

- Insomnia - A variety of mind-body therapies (e.g., relaxation techniques; meditation; biofeedback) may help to improve the quality of sleep of cancer patients who experience insomnia.

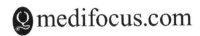

Dietary Modification and Supplementation

Evidence from epidemiological studies strongly supports a relationship between dietary factors and the risk for developing certain types of cancers. In general, a diet that is rich in certain food constituents (e.g., fruits, vegetable, fiber) appears to be protective against the development of cancer. In contrast, excessive consumption of other dietary substances (e.g., animal fats, alcohol) appears to increase the risk of certain types of cancers. Some vitamins that possess antioxidant properties (e.g., vitamins A, C, and E) may protect against certain types of cancers by protecting the body's cells from damage by certain compounds known as *free radicals*.

The role of dietary modification and antioxidant vitamin supplementation in slowing the progression of cancer continues to be an area of ongoing research. Currently, there are no conclusive studies which prove that any type of dietary modification or antioxidant vitamin supplementation can alter the progression of the disease in cancer patients.

Cancer patients who are considering dietary modification and/or antioxidant vitamin supplementation need to be aware of certain risks that may be associated with these regimens:

- Unintentional weight loss is a relatively common side-effect of cancer treatment, particularly among patients who are undergoing chemotherapy and/or radiation therapy. Excessive reduction of certain dietary components, such as dietary fat intake, may increase the risk of malnutrition in cancer patients. It is, therefore, important for patients to discuss the potential risks and benefits of any dietary modification with their oncologist before making a decision to modify their dietary intake.

- Some radical dietary regimens, such as *macrobiotic diets* (that are primarily vegetarian) may potentially promote the progression of disease in women with estrogen-receptor positive breast cancer or endometrial cancer due to their high content of isoflavonoid phytoestrogens. The same concern applies to diets that promote soy supplementation as a means of slowing the progression of cancer. Soy products contain high amounts of isoflavonoid phytoestrogens and should be avoided by women with estrogen-receptor positive tumors.

- High doses of certain antioxidant vitamin supplements (vitamins C and E) may increase the risk of bleeding complications in patients who have low levels of platelets in the bloodstream (thrombocytopenia) or patients who are taking

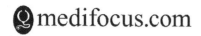
anticoagulant medications. High doses of vitamin A can cause a condition called *Hypervitaminosis A* (Vitamin A toxicity) that can cause symptoms such as nausea, vomiting, headaches, blurry vision, and impaired consciousness.

Herbal Products

Currently there is a lack of sufficient scientific evidence to recommend the use of herbal products or supplements for the treatment of cancer. The safety of herbal formulations and products is also a major factor that should be taken into consideration by consumers. The National Center for Complementary and Alternative Medicine (NCCAM) urges consumers to be aware of several important safety issues pertaining to herbal products and supplements, including:

- Do not necessarily assume that just because many of these products are labeled as "natural", they are completely safe and, therefore, cannot cause potentially serious adverse reactions. If you have any concerns about the possible side-effects of a particular herbal product or supplement, ask a pharmacist or your doctor about possible side-effects or interactions with other medications that you may be taking.

- Women who are pregnant or who are nursing should be especially cautious about using herbal products and supplements since the safety of many of these products has not established for use during pregnancy or lactation.

- Find out as much information as you can about a particular herbal product you are considering before taking it. If you have concerns or questions about a product, speak to a health care professional and get their advice. Moreover, you should always only use these products under the guidance of a health care professional.

- Some herbal products and supplements may interact with other medications that you may be taking and may cause adverse side-effects. Some herbal products may interfere with the action of certain chemotherapeutic agents that are used in the treatment of cancer. It is, therefore, important to notify your doctor about any herbal products you may be using or are considering using in order to prevent or reduce the possibility of adverse herb/drug interactions.

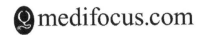

Quality of Life Issues in Cancer

The diagnosis of any type of cancer is a frightening, life-altering event for both the patient and their family. The potential for a diminished quality of life for newly diagnosed cancer patients becomes an immediate, pressing concern when confronted with anxiety, fear, pain, the prospect of a long course of treatments that may cause significant side effects, and the possibility that the treatments may not work. It is critically important, however, for cancer patients and their families to address and learn to cope with the physical, emotional, and social issues that, if ignored and left to "fester", can rapidly lead to a significantly reduced quality of life.

Over the years, cancer specialists and other allied health-care professionals have come to realize that addressing a cancer patient's quality of life issues is an integral component of a comprehensive, overall cancer treatment strategy. From a practical perspective, that means developing an effective treatment plan that aims not only to control and/or to eradicate the patient's cancer with medical and/or surgical therapy but, at the same time, also takes into consideration critical issues of supportive care throughout the course of treatment and offers the patient the best chances of maintaining a reasonably high level quality of life. In fact, most cancer specialists now consider supportive care as an essential component of an overall, effective cancer treatment plan.

Factors Affecting Quality of Life in Cancer Patients

Cancer patients are confronted with a variety of physical, emotional, and social issues that, if left unchecked or ignored, can rapidly contribute to a diminished quality of life. In general, some of the more common problems encountered by cancer patients either as a result of the disease itself or as a side-effect of cancer treatments include:

- Sleep disorders
- Fatigue
- Diminished exercise capacity
- Unintentional weight loss
- Psychological stress
- Cancer-related pain

Sleep Disorders
Lack of adequate sleep due to anxiety, stress, pain, or treatment side-effects can lead to severe daytime fatigue that, in turn, can interfere with the ability to function and perform routine activities of daily living. Perhaps now, more than ever before, getting an adequate amount of sleep is critical to enable the body and mind to cope with the additional physical

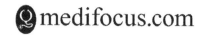

and emotional burdens resulting from cancer and its treatment. If sleep disturbances begin to affect your functional ability and diminish your quality of life, a variety of options are available to deal with the problem. These treatment options include learning new sleep habits (improved sleep hygiene practices); complementary therapies (e.g., relaxation techniques, biofeedback, meditation); and the use of prescription sleep medications. If lack of sleep is affecting your quality of life and interfering with your activities of daily living, talk with your doctor about developing an individualized treatment plan to help improve your quality of sleep.

Fatigue

Fatigue is perhaps the most common and potentially debilitating symptom experienced by cancer patients that can have a significant negative impact on routine activities of daily living and diminish quality of life. Fatigue may be attributed to a variety of causes including side-effects of cancer treatments (e.g., chemotherapy, radiation therapy), anemia, sleep deprivation resulting from insomnia, chronic pain, inadequate nutrition, and lack of physical exercise. In many cases, a combination of factors contributes to fatigue, exhaustion, and a general lack of energy. It is important to notify your cancer specialist or primary health care provider if you begin to experience bouts of fatigue lasting a few days or longer.

A variety of strategies are available to overcome the problem of fatigue in cancer patients. Fatigue related to anemia (low numbers of red blood cells) can be treated with blood transfusions and drugs, such as *erythropoietin* (e.g., Procrit) that promote the production of red blood cells. Fatigue not related to anemia may be managed with lifestyle modifications such as proper nutrition, regular exercise, and improved sleep hygiene practices.

Exercise

In the past, cancer patients were usually advised to "relax", "take it easy" and "don't overdo it". More recently, however, doctors are beginning to realize the potential benefits of physical exercise for cancer patients undergoing treatment as well as for cancer survivors. Researchers are continuing to explore the effect of physical exercise on survival rates for various types of cancers. In general, the potential benefits of physical activity for patients suffering from chronic diseases include enhanced physical and mental function and improved quality of life. For cancer patients, the potential benefits of exercise also include decreased fatigue, improved appetite, better toleration of side effects of chemotherapy and radiation therapy, and improved quality of life.

It is important to speak to your cancer specialist about the types of exercise that may be appropriate at various stages of your cancer treatment and the types of physical activities that you should avoid.

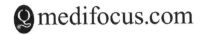 **medifocus.com**

Unintentional Weight Loss

One of the most common symptoms experienced by cancer patients is *unintentional weight loss* which can lead to malnutrition, increased susceptibility to infections, reduced quality of life, and shorter survival time. The underlying causes of unintentional weight loss in cancer patients may be attributed to a variety of factors including loss of appetite associated with chemotherapy and/or radiation therapy and psychological disturbances such as depression which has been found to affect up to 25% of cancer patients.

From a metabolic perspective, unintentional weight loss may be understood by the increased energy (calories) required by cancer cells to grow and spread as well as the increased energy requirements of the body to mount an effective response to fight the cancer. A net loss in weight occurs when the body uses more calories from stored energy reserves than is available from calories ingested from nutrients in the diet. Metabolic changes in cancer can also cause a condition called *cachexia* - a generalized wasting condition involving the loss of muscle mass and fat. Cachexia may develop even in people with good nutritional intake due to the failure of the body to absorb nutrients. Symptoms of cachexia, which affects about 50% of all cancer patients, include loss of appetite, weight loss, wasting of muscle mass, generalized fatigue, and significantly reduced capacity to perform routine activities of daily living.

The management of weight loss in cancer patients usually involves nutritional counseling to ensure an adequate intake of calories. Nutritional counseling can also help cancer patients develop new eating habits to prevent further weight loss including eating foods that are rich in calories or protein; eating smaller meals more frequently throughout the course of the day; "snacking" between meals; and drinking high-calorie liquid nutritional supplements (e.g., Boost, Ensure, Sustacal). In some cases, medications such as megestrol acetate (Megace) or dexamethasone (Decadron) may be prescribed to stimulate the appetite.

Your cancer specialist, working together with a nutritionist and a dietician, can help you develop and maintain a well-balanced diet to ensure that your body receives an adequate level of nutrition not only during the course of your cancer treatments but also during the recovery phase.

Psychological Stress

The diagnosis of cancer is a life-altering event that may evoke feelings of anxiety, fear, depression, hopelessness, and severe psychological stress in many patients. Studies have shown that about 25% of cancer patients suffer from depression. Conventional treatments for anxiety, stress, and depression may involve the administration of prescription anti-anxiety medications or antidepressants which may cause undesirable side-effects in some patients. Specific types of *psychotherapy* or "talk therapy" can also help relieve

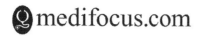

depression in cancer patients.

Studies have shown that a variety of complementary and alternative medicine (CAM) therapies are useful for controlling anxiety and other mood disturbances when used in conjunction with conventional treatments. These include:

- Mind-body interventions - relaxation techniques, guided-imagery, meditation, hypnosis
- Acupuncture
- Massage therapy
- Music therapy

In general, patients with severe mood disturbances (e.g., panic attacks; suicide ideation) require immediate psychological evaluation and treatment to stabilize their acute condition before CAM therapies may be considered. For most patients with mild to moderate anxiety and mood disturbances, CAM therapies are a useful adjunct to conventional treatments for managing psychological distress. Techniques such as mind-body interventions, acupuncture, and music therapy are generally safe when performed by qualified, experienced practitioners and can help cancer patients better cope with feelings of anxiety, fear, hopelessness, and depression. Although some herbs and dietary supplements (e.g., Kava Kava; St. John's Wort; Passionflower) have been reported to relieve anxiety and mood disturbances, some experts have discouraged the use of these products in cancer patients because they may interfere with drugs used to treat cancer (chemotherapeutic agents) and/or other medications that patients may be taking. Patients should discuss the risks and benefits of using any herbal medications/dietary supplements with their oncologist before taking any of these products, particularly if they are undergoing chemotherapy, radiation therapy, or surgery.

Cancer-Related Pain

Pain is a relatively common symptom that is experienced by many cancer patients. In recent years, increased awareness about this problem has led to important advances in the management of patients with cancer-related pain. In fact, today most major cancer centers in the United States have established pain management clinics, usually located within the Anesthesiology department of a hospital, that specialize in helping patients to better control their cancer-related pain.

Most often, the source of cancer-related pain is the tumor itself. This can occur when a tumor spreads and invades other tissues or organs of the body; when a tumor compresses a nearby nerve or the spinal cord; or when a tumor causes intestinal obstruction. Cancer-related pain may also be caused by some procedures that are used for the diagnosis and treatment of cancer. Examples include tissue biopsy; placement of a central line catheter; bone marrow aspiration; and spinal tap.

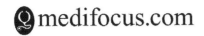
Irrespective of the source of your cancer pain, it is important to notify your oncologist or primary care doctor about any pain or discomfort that you may be experiencing so that appropriate measures can be taken to eliminate or better control the pain. In developing an individualized pain control strategy, your doctor will want to learn as much as possible about the pain you are experiencing, including:

- When did the pain start?
- How long does the pain last (acute or chronic)?
- Is the pain minor, moderate, or severe?
- Is the pain localized to a particular area of the body?
- Are there any specific activities or events that either "trigger" the pain or help to alleviate the pain?
- To what extent does the pain interfere with your quality of life and activities of daily living?
- Are you currently taking any pain medications?

Drug Therapy for Cancer-Related Pain

A wide range of pain medications is available for helping patients better cope with cancer-related pain. Your doctor will determine the specific type of medication that is most suitable for you based on the information you provide including the severity of the pain (e.g., mild, moderate, or severe) and the duration of the pain. You can help your doctor in selecting the most appropriate pain medication for your specific type of cancer pain by providing him/her with as much information as possible about the nature and characteristics of the pain. Be sure to also notify your doctor if:

- You are allergic to any medications
- You have previously experienced any serious side-effects from pain medications (e.g., gastrointestinal bleeding)
- You have a current or past history of stomach ulcers
- You are taking any other pain medications including herbal products or medications.

In general, the following pain medication treatment options are available in the management of cancer-related pain based upon the severity of the pain:

- Non-Steroidal Anti-Inflammatory Drugs - Mild cancer-related pain can usually be managed with a variety of pain medications that belong to the general family of drugs known as *non-steroidal anti-inflammatory drugs* (NSAIDs). Examples of NSAIDs that are available "over-the-counter" include:

  - aspirin (e.g., Bayer)
  - acetaminophen (e.g., Tylenol)

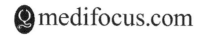
- ibuprofen (e.g., Motrin)
- naproxen (e.g., Aleve)

Some NSAIDs used for the treatment of pain, including cancer-related pain, are available by prescription only. Examples include diclofenac (e.g., Voltaren); indomethacin (Indocin); ketoprofen (e.g., Orudis); and Cox-2 inhibitors (e.g., Celebrex), among others.

- Narcotic (Opioid) Analgesics - If you are experiencing mild to moderate cancer-related pain, your doctor may prescribe a medication that belongs to a family of drugs known as *narcotic analgesics*. Examples include:

  - codeine
  - morphine
  - buprenorphine (e.g., Subutex; Suboxone)
  - fentanyl (e.g., Duragesic)
  - oxycodone (e.g., OxyNorm; OxyContin)
  - hydrocodone (e.g., Vicodin; Lortab)
  - hydromorphone (e.g., Dilaudid)

In some cases, combination pain medication tablets containing an NSAID plus a narcotic analgesic may be prescribed for the management of mild to moderate cancer-related pain. Examples of combination pain medication tablets include Percodan (aspirin plus oxycodone); Percocet (acetaminophen plus oxycodone); Co-codamol (acetaminophen plus codeine); and Co-codaprin (aspirin plus codeine)

As a general "rule of thumb", cancer patients with mild to moderate pain are usually started on "weaker" opioid-based medications (e.g., codeine) and, if necessary, are switched to stronger opioid medications (e.g., fentanyl, oxycodone, morphine).

Common side-effects of narcotic analgesics include constipation, lethargy, drowsiness, nausea/vomiting, and sleepiness. In addition, a major concern with the use of narcotic analgesics is the possibility of addiction to the medications. Be sure you notify your doctor if you have a current or past history of drug and/or alcohol abuse before taking narcotic analgesics. Also speak with your doctor about strategies that can be used to manage the side-effects of narcotic analgesics. For example, constipation may be managed by taking a stool softener (e.g., Colace; Senokot). If you experience drowsiness or sleepiness when you take your pain medication, you should avoid any activities that may pose a danger to yourself or others (e.g., driving a car; mowing the lawn).

- Adjuvant Pain Medications - Some drugs that are primary used to treat conditions other than pain also possess analgesic (pain-relieving) properties. These drugs are known as *adjuvant pain medications* and are sometimes prescribed, alone or in combination with other medications, for the management of cancer-related pain. Examples include:

- anticonvulsants - This class of drugs is used primarily to treat seizures. Examples of anticonvulsants that may also be used to treat cancer pain include: gabapentin (e.g.,Neurontin); carbamazepine (e.g., Tegretol); phenytoin (e.g., Dilantin); and topiramate (e.g., Topamax)

- antidepressants - This class of drugs is used primarily to treat depression. Examples of antidepressants that may be also be used to treat cancer pain include: amitriptylene (e.g., Elavil); desipramine (e.g., Norpramin); doxepin (e.g., Sinequon); and impipramine (e.g., Tofranil).

- bisphosphonates - This class of drugs is used primarily for the treatment of osteoporosis. Studies have also demonstrated that bisphosphonates may relieve bone pain in cancer patients. Examples include: alendronate (e.g., Fosamax); pamidronate (Aredia); and etidronate (e.g., Didronel).

- corticosteroids - This class of drugs is used primarily to treat inflammatory conditions such as rheumatoid arthritis, osteoarthritis, and ankylosing spondylitis. By reducing inflammation, corticosteroids also reduce pain. A common type of corticosteroid drug used for the management of cancer pain is dexamethasone (e.g., Dexmethsone).

- Breakthrough Cancer Pain - Despite the regular use of pain medications on a fixed schedule, many cancer patients (estimates range from 50% to 65%) experience a type of pain known as *breakthrough cancer pain*. This type of pain is characterized by a sudden onset, may last from minutes to hours, and is usually severe in nature. Breakthrough cancer pain occurs most often in patients who are experiencing persistent or chronic cancer pain who notice a sudden, periodic "flare-up" of severe pain even though they are taking pain medication on a regular schedule.

Breakthrough cancer pain is most often treated with opioid medications that act quickly, such as immediate release morphine tablets or capsules, but are rapidly eliminated from the body so that they cause less side-effects. The U.S. Food and Drug Administration (FDA) has also approved a drug called ACTIQ (Oral Transmucosal Fentanyl Citrate) in the form of a lozenge on a stick that dissolves slowly in the mouth for the treatment of breakthrough cancer pain. Be sure to notify your doctor if you think you may be experiencing

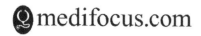

breakthrough pain that is not controlled with your regular fixed-schedule pain medications so that he/she may determine the best course of treatment to alleviate your pain.

For more information about cancer-related pain and the treatment options, please click on the following link: http://www.cancer-pain.org

The Role of Complementary and Alternative Medicine Therapies in Cancer-Related Pain

As a general rule, complementary and alternative medicine (CAM) therapies are usually not considered as a viable treatment option for the management of acute cancer-related pain. Acute cancer-related pain usually responds best to conventional drug therapy (e.g., NSAIDs; narcotic analgesics; adjuvant pain medications). Surgery may also be necessary for the treatment of some types of acute cancer pain such as when a tumor compresses a nearby nerve or the spinal cord or if the tumor is causing abdominal or intestinal obstruction. Once the acute pain has been brought under control by conventional treatment modalities, CAM therapies may be considered in the management of *chronic* (persistent) cancer-related pain. A potential benefit of using CAM therapies in conjunction with conventional treatments for the management of chronic cancer-related pain is that they may reduce the dosage of conventional pain medications that may be required to achieve chronic pain control and, therefore, also potentially reduce the side-effects that may be associated with conventional pain medications.

A variety of CAM therapies, when used in conjunction with conventional treatments, may be beneficial for the management of chronic cancer-related pain, including:

- Meditation
- Guided imagery
- Hypnosis
- Relaxation techniques
- Massage therapy
- Reflexology
- Acupuncture
- Yoga
- Aromatherapy

Where Can You Find Supportive Care?

Fortunately, supportive care is available for cancer patients and their families from a multitude of resources. These include:

- Cancer Centers - the hospital or cancer center where you have chosen to receive your treatment is an excellent starting point in your search for supportive cancer care. Many major hospitals and comprehensive cancer centers provide access to a variety of resources for cancer patients including educational, psychological, and social services support.

- Your Cancer Physician - the primary cancer specialist who is in charge of your care and is responsible for your overall treatment is also an excellent resource of information and support. These cancer specialists are in the business of caring for cancer patients and usually have a wealth of knowledge about the physical, psychological, and social issues confronting patients who have been diagnosed with cancer. Depending upon your specific type of cancer, a variety of cancer specialists may be involved in your treatment including an:

  - oncologist
  - hematologist
  - radiation oncologist
  - surgical oncologist

- Oncology Nurses - if your treatment plan includes chemotherapy, you will be assigned a nurse oncologist who will administer your drugs and monitor side-effects or other problems that may occur during your chemotherapy sessions. Nurse oncologists are highly trained professionals who are a wonderful source of information and can provide educational materials, emotional support, and practical tips for dealing with adverse side-effects of chemotherapy such as nausea, fatigue, and pain.

- Your Primary Care Physician - it is likely that a visit to your primary care physician led to the discovery and diagnosis of your cancer and that your primary care physician referred you to a cancer specialist for treatment. Your primary care physician will usually work closely with your cancer specialist in following your progress both during as well as after treatment has been completed. It is important to be open and frank with your primary care physician and talk to him/her about any physical or emotional problems that you may experience so that they can help you get over these difficult periods.

- Nurse Practitioners - Nurse practitioners are registered nurses (RNs) who have completed additional courses and training. They can work with or without the supervision of a physician. Their scope of work includes both diagnosis and treatment of diseases and, in many states, they can also write prescriptions.

- Physician's Assistants - A physician's assistant is a licensed health care professional who provides care under the supervision of a physician. Physician's assistants

ⓠmedifocus.com

provide a broad range of diagnostic and therapeutic services including ordering and interpreting laboratory tests, diagnosing and treating diseases and conditions, conducting physical examinations, and assisting in surgery.

- Nutritionists/Dieticians - consultation with a nutritional expert can help ensure that you maintain an adequate level of nutrition throughout your cancer treatment and that your body has sufficient energy to withstand the rigorous cancer treatments which may carry significant side-effects. Well-nourished cancer patients also have more energy and are less prone to experience severe fatigue and exhaustion.

- Social Workers - a social worker who is experienced in working with cancer patients (oncology social workers) can provide valuable assistance in dealing with a variety of social and emotional issues including:

  - teaching patients and families to navigate the complexities of the health-care system
  - helping with financial and health insurance issues
  - assisting family members in adjusting to new roles and responsibilities
  - arranging home health care for patients requiring home-based treatments
  - providing access to local, state, and government agencies that provide social and health services
  - helping cancer patients deal with employees and return to work issues

- Mental Health Professionals - A psychiatrist or psychologist with expertise in diagnosing and treating psychological and emotional disturbances in cancer patients (e.g., anxiety, fear, depression, self-image issues) is an integral member of the comprehensive cancer team who can help patients better cope and adjust to living with cancer.

- Clergy - a trusted member of the clergy can provide spiritual guidance, reassurance, and hope to cancer patients and their families.

- Sex Therapists - a sex therapist can help cancer patients who experience a reduced libido or other sexual problems that may develop as a consequence of the cancer itself or treatment related side-effects.

- Family and Friends - family, friends, and long-term acquaintances who know you best are one of your most important support networks and can provide emotional support, guidance, and encouragement both during and long after you've completed your course of cancer therapy. Now, more than ever, you need to open-up to your family and friends and share your feelings, fears, and emotions with them. They will appreciate your willingness to trust and confide in them and you will benefit from

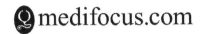

their reassurance, encouragement, positive attitude, and continuous love.

- Organizations and Support Groups - a broad range of organizations and support groups that specialize in helping cancer patients and their families represent a valuable source of support, networking, access to services, and for obtaining important educational cancer materials. Some of these major organizations may be located in your city and some cancer support groups may even have branches in your neighborhood. Joining a cancer support group may be one of the most important steps you take to help yourself on the road to recovery. Networking and "connecting" with other cancer patients and cancer survivors who understand and share your fears and concerns can be an important source of consolation, comfort, and peace of mind knowing that you are not alone in this battle. Other cancer patients have been down this road before and learning about their personal experiences and coping strategies can help you work your way through this difficult period in your life.

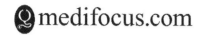 medifocus.com

- What is the grade of my lymphoma (low-, intermediate-, or high-grade)?
- What is the stage of my lymphoma (Stage I, II, IV, or IV)?
- Is my lymphoma localized to the lymph nodes or has it spread to any other areas of the body?
- What treatments do you recommend for my type of lymphoma?
- What are my treatment options?
- What are the risks and benefits of each type of treatment?
- What is the prognosis for my type of lymphoma based on the International Prognostic Index scoring system?
- What kind of support do you provide for lymphoma patients?
- Are there any clinical trials in which I may be eligible to participate?
- Information about clinical trials can be found at the Centerwatch Clinical Trials Listing Service web site at http://www.centerwatch.com.

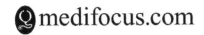

NOTES

Use this page for taking notes as you review your Guidebook

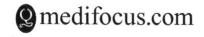

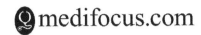 medifocus.com

3 - Guide to the Medical Literature

Introduction

This section of your *MediFocus Guidebook* is a comprehensive bibliography of important recent medical literature published about the condition from authoritative, trustworthy medical journals. This is the same information that is used by physicians and researchers to keep up with the latest advances in clinical medicine and biomedical research. A broad spectrum of articles is included in each *MediFocus Guidebook* to provide information about standard treatments, treatment options, new developments, and advances in research.

To facilitate your review and analysis of this information, the articles in this *MediFocus Guidebook* are grouped in the following categories:

- Review Articles - 60 Articles
- General Interest Articles - 51 Articles
- Drug Therapy Articles - 21 Articles
- Clinical Trials Articles - 69 Articles
- Radiation Therapy Articles - 3 Articles
- Stem Cell Transplantation Articles - 15 Articles
- Radioimmunotherapy Articles - 5 Articles

The following information is provided for each of the articles referenced in this section of your *MediFocus Guidebook:*

- Title of the article
- Name of the authors
- Institution where the study was done
- Journal reference (Volume, page numbers, year of publication)
- Link to Abstract (brief summary of the actual article)

Linking to Abstracts: Most of the medical journal articles referenced in this section of your *MediFocus Guidebook* include an abstract (brief summary of the actual article) that can be accessed online via the National Library of Medicine's PubMed® database. You can easily access the individual article abstracts online by entering the individual URL address for a particular article into your web browser, or by going to the following special URL:

http://www.medifocus.com/links/HM009/0212

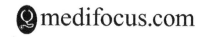

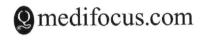

Recent Literature: What Your Doctor Reads

Database: PubMed <January 2007 to January 2012>

Review Articles

1.

Ofatumumab in the treatment of low-grade non-Hodgkin's lymphomas and chronic lymphocytic leukemia.

Authors: Bello C; Veliz M; Pinilla-Ibarz J
Institution: H Lee Moffitt Cancer, 12901 Magnolia Drive, FOB3, Tampa, FL 33612, USA. celeste.bello@moffitt.org
Journal: Expert Rev Clin Immunol. 2011 May;7(3):295-300.
Abstract Link: http://www.medifocus.com/abstracts.php?gid=HM009&ID=21595596

2.

Primary gastrointestinal lymphoma.

Authors: Ghimire P; Wu GY; Zhu L
Institution: Department of Magnetic Resonance Imaging, Zhongnan Hospital, Wuhan University, 169 East Lake Road, Wuhan 430071, Hubei Province, China.
Journal: World J Gastroenterol. 2011 Feb 14;17(6):697-707.
Abstract Link: http://www.medifocus.com/abstracts.php?gid=HM009&ID=21390139

3.

Pharmacotherapy for primary CNS lymphoma: progress beyond methotrexate?

Authors: Graber JJ; Omuro A
Institution: Department of Neurology, Memorial Sloan-Kettering Cancer Center, New York, New York, USA.
Journal: CNS Drugs. 2011 Jun 1;25(6):447-57. doi: 10.2165/11589030-000000000-00000.
Abstract Link: http://www.medifocus.com/abstracts.php?gid=HM009&ID=21649446

Go to http://www.medifocus.com/links/HM009/0212 for direct online access to the above Abstract Links.

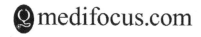

4.

Stem cell transplantation for indolent lymphoma and chronic lymphocytic leukemia.

Authors: Gribben JG; Hosing C; Maloney DG

Institution: Barts and The London School of Medicine, London, United Kingdom. j.gribben@qmul.ac.uk

Journal: Biol Blood Marrow Transplant. 2011 Jan;17(1 Suppl):S63-70.

Abstract Link: http://www.medifocus.com/abstracts.php?gid=HM009&ID=21195313

5.

Chemotherapy and antibody combinations for relapsed/refractory non-Hodgkin's lymphoma.

Authors: Halwani AS; Link BK

Institution: Department of Medicine, University of Iowa College of Medicine, Holden Comprehensive Cancer Center, 200 Hawkins Drive, Iowa City, IA 52242, USA.

Journal: Expert Rev Anticancer Ther. 2011 Mar;11(3):443-55.

Abstract Link: http://www.medifocus.com/abstracts.php?gid=HM009&ID=21417857

6.

Stem-cell transplantation in T-cell non-Hodgkin's lymphomas.

Authors: Hosing C; Champlin RE

Institution: Department of Stem Cell Transplantation and Cellular Therapy, The University of Texas MD Anderson Cancer Center, Houston, TX 77030, USA.

Journal: Ann Oncol. 2011 Jul;22(7):1471-7. Epub 2011 May 5.

Abstract Link: http://www.medifocus.com/abstracts.php?gid=HM009&ID=21551006

Go to http://www.medifocus.com/links/HM009/0212 for direct online access to the above Abstract Links.

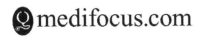

7.

Novel therapeutics for aggressive non-Hodgkin's lymphoma.

Authors:	Mahadevan D; Fisher RI
Institution:	Arizona Cancer Center, Tucson, AZ, USA. dmahadevan@azcc.arizona.edu
Journal:	J Clin Oncol. 2011 May 10;29(14):1876-84. Epub 2011 Apr 11.
Abstract Link:	http://www.medifocus.com/abstracts.php?gid=HM009&ID=21483007

8.

New antibody drug treatments for lymphoma.

Authors:	Mayes S; Brown N; Illidge TM
Institution:	University of Manchester, Manchester Academic Health Science Centre, School of Cancer and Enabling Sciences, School of Medicine, Manchester, M20 4BX, UK.
Journal:	Expert Opin Biol Ther. 2011 May;11(5):623-40. Epub 2011 Mar 14.
Abstract Link:	http://www.medifocus.com/abstracts.php?gid=HM009&ID=21395497

9.

Current standards and future strategies in immunochemotherapy of non-Hodgkin's lymphoma.

Authors:	Motta G; Cea M; Carbone F; Augusti V; Moran E; Patrone F; Nencioni A
Institution:	Department of Internal Medicine, University of Genoa, Genoa, Italy.
Journal:	J BUON. 2011 Jan-Mar;16(1):9-15.
Abstract Link:	http://www.medifocus.com/abstracts.php?gid=HM009&ID=21674844

Go to http://www.medifocus.com/links/HM009/0212 for direct online access to the above Abstract Links.

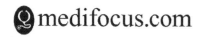

10.

The impact of treatment, socio-demographic and clinical characteristics on health-related quality of life among Hodgkin's and non-Hodgkin's lymphoma survivors: a systematic review.

Authors: Oerlemans S; Mols F; Nijziel MR; Lybeert M; van de Poll-Franse LV

Institution: Research Department, Comprehensive Cancer Centre South, Eindhoven, The Netherlands. s.oerlemans@ikz.nl

Journal: Ann Hematol. 2011 Sep;90(9):993-1004. Epub 2011 Jun 14.

Abstract Link: http://www.medifocus.com/abstracts.php?gid=HM009&ID=21670973

11.

New therapeutic targets and drugs in non-Hodgkin's lymphoma.

Authors: Sawas A; Diefenbach C; O'Connor OA

Institution: NYU Cancer Institute, School of Medicine, NYU Langone Medical Center, New York, New York 10016, USA.

Journal: Curr Opin Hematol. 2011 Jul;18(4):280-7.

Abstract Link: http://www.medifocus.com/abstracts.php?gid=HM009&ID=21654386

12.

Current status of allogeneic transplantation for aggressive non-Hodgkin lymphoma.

Author: van Besien K

Institution: Stem Cell Transplant Program, University of Chicago, Chicago, Illinois, USA.

Journal: Curr Opin Oncol. 2011 Nov;23(6):681-91.

Abstract Link: http://www.medifocus.com/abstracts.php?gid=HM009&ID=21946246

Go to http://www.medifocus.com/links/HM009/0212 for direct online access to the above Abstract Links.

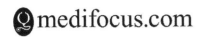
13.

Radioimmunotherapy for the treatment of non-Hodgkin lymphoma: current status and future applications.

Authors:	Ahmed S; Winter JN; Gordon LI; Evens AM
Institution:	Division of Hematology/Oncology, Northwestern University Feinberg School of Medicine, Chicago, IL, USA.
Journal:	Leuk Lymphoma. 2010 Jul;51(7):1163-77.
Abstract Link:	http://www.medifocus.com/abstracts.php?gid=HM009&ID=20470217

14.

Galiximab: a review.

Authors:	Bhat S; Czuczman MS
Institution:	Roswell Park Cancer Institute, Elm and Carlton Streets, Buffalo, NY 14263, USA.
Journal:	Expert Opin Biol Ther. 2010 Mar;10(3):451-8.
Abstract Link:	http://www.medifocus.com/abstracts.php?gid=HM009&ID=20092425

15.

Optimal use of bendamustine in chronic lymphocytic leukemia, non-Hodgkin lymphomas, and multiple myeloma: treatment recommendations from an international consensus panel.

Authors:	Cheson BD; Wendtner CM; Pieper A; Dreyling M; Friedberg J; Hoelzer D; Moreau P; Gribben J; Knop S; Montillo M; Rummel M
Institution:	Division of Hematology-Oncology, Georgetown University Hospital, Lombardi Comprehensive Cancer Center, Washington, DC 20007, USA. bdc4@georgetown.edu
Journal:	Clin Lymphoma Myeloma Leuk. 2010 Feb;10(1):21-7.
Abstract Link:	http://www.medifocus.com/abstracts.php?gid=HM009&ID=20223726

Go to http://www.medifocus.com/links/HM009/0212 for direct online access to the above Abstract Links.

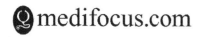
medifocus.com

16.

Plerixafor for stem cell mobilization in patients with non-Hodgkin's lymphoma and multiple myeloma.

Authors: Choi HY; Yong CS; Yoo BK

Institution: College of Pharmacy, Yeungnam University, Gyeongsan, Kyungbuk, Korea.

Journal: Ann Pharmacother. 2010 Jan;44(1):117-26. Epub 2009 Dec 15.

Abstract Link: http://www.medifocus.com/abstracts.php?gid=HM009&ID=20009003

17.

Bendamustine for the treatment of indolent non-Hodgkin's lymphoma and chronic lymphocytic leukemia.

Authors: Elefante A; Czuczman MS

Institution: Department of Pharmacy, Roswell Park Cancer Institute, Elm and Carlton Streets, Buffalo, NY 14263, USA. angie.elefante@roswellpark.org

Journal: Am J Health Syst Pharm. 2010 May 1;67(9):713-23.

Abstract Link: http://www.medifocus.com/abstracts.php?gid=HM009&ID=20410545

18.

Bendamustine: a review of its use in the management of indolent non-Hodgkin's lymphoma and mantle cell lymphoma.

Author: Garnock-Jones KP

Institution: Adis, a Wolters Kluwer Business, Auckland, New Zealand. demail@adis.co.nz

Journal: Drugs. 2010 Sep 10;70(13):1703-18. doi: 10.2165/11205860-000000000-00000.

Abstract Link: http://www.medifocus.com/abstracts.php?gid=HM009&ID=20731477

Go to http://www.medifocus.com/links/HM009/0212 for direct online access to the above Abstract Links.

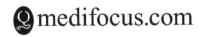
19.

Primary central nervous system lymphoma.

Authors:	Gerstner ER; Batchelor TT
Institution:	Division of Hematology and Oncology, Massachusetts General Hospital Cancer Center and Harvard Medical School, Boston, MA, USA. egerstner@partners.org
Journal:	Arch Neurol. 2010 Mar;67(3):291-7.
Abstract Link:	http://www.medifocus.com/abstracts.php?gid=HM009&ID=20212226

20.

Emerging non-transplant-based strategies in treating pediatric non-Hodgkin's lymphoma.

Authors:	Gore L; Trippett TM
Institution:	Center for Cancer and Blood Disorders, The Children's Hospital, The University of Colorado Cancer Center, Denver, 80045, USA. lia.gore@ucdenver.edu
Journal:	Curr Hematol Malig Rep. 2010 Oct;5(4):177-84.
Abstract Link:	http://www.medifocus.com/abstracts.php?gid=HM009&ID=20640605

21.

Maintenance and consolidation strategies in non-Hodgkin's lymphoma: A review of the data.

Author:	Hagemeister FB
Institution:	Department of Lymphoma/Myeloma, M. D. Anderson Cancer Center, Houston, TX 77030, USA. fhagemei@mdanderson.org
Journal:	Curr Oncol Rep. 2010 Nov;12(6):395-401.
Abstract Link:	http://www.medifocus.com/abstracts.php?gid=HM009&ID=20820960

Go to http://www.medifocus.com/links/HM009/0212 for direct online access to the above Abstract Links.

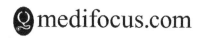

22.

Benzene and the risk of non-Hodgkin lymphoma: a review and meta-analysis of the literature.

Authors:	Kane EV; Newton R
Institution:	Epidemiology and Genetics Unit, Department of Health Sciences, Seebohm Rowntree Building, University of York, YO10 5DD, UK. eleanor.kane@egu.york.ac.uk <eleanor.kane@egu.york.ac.uk>
Journal:	Cancer Epidemiol. 2010 Feb;34(1):7-12. Epub 2010 Jan 13.
Abstract Link:	http://www.medifocus.com/abstracts.php?gid=HM009&ID=20075019

23.

Diversity in antibody-based approaches to non-Hodgkin lymphoma.

Authors:	Maloney D; Morschhauser F; Linden O; Hagenbeek A; Gisselbrecht C
Institution:	Fred Hutchinson Cancer Research Center, Division of Oncology, University of Washington, Seattle, USA.
Journal:	Leuk Lymphoma. 2010 Aug;51 Suppl 1:20-7.
Abstract Link:	http://www.medifocus.com/abstracts.php?gid=HM009&ID=20815760

24.

Monoclonal antibodies for non-Hodgkin's lymphoma: state of the art and perspectives.

Authors:	Motta G; Cea M; Moran E; Carbone F; Augusti V; Patrone F; Nencioni A
Institution:	Department of Internal Medicine, University of Genoa, Room 221, V.le Benedetto XV 6, 16132 Genoa, Italy.
Journal:	Clin Dev Immunol. 2010;2010:428253. Epub 2011 Mar 6.
Abstract Link:	http://www.medifocus.com/abstracts.php?gid=HM009&ID=21437222

Go to http://www.medifocus.com/links/HM009/0212 for direct online access to the above Abstract Links.

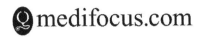

25.

Pixantrone for the treatment of aggressive non-Hodgkin lymphoma.

Authors: Mukherji D; Pettengell R

Institution: St Georges Hospital, Blackshaw Road, Tooting, London SW170QT, UK.

Journal: Expert Opin Pharmacother. 2010 Aug;11(11):1915-23.

Abstract Link: http://www.medifocus.com/abstracts.php?gid=HM009&ID=20569087

26.

Stem cell transplantation in childhood non-Hodgkin's lymphomas.

Authors: Okur FV; Krance R

Institution: Texas Children's Cancer Center, Houston, TX 77030, USA. fvokur@txccc.org

Journal: Curr Hematol Malig Rep. 2010 Oct;5(4):192-9.

Abstract Link: http://www.medifocus.com/abstracts.php?gid=HM009&ID=20661786

27.

Improving the efficacy of radioimmunotherapy for non-Hodgkin lymphomas.

Authors: Palanca-Wessels MC; Press OW

Institution: Division of Hematology, Department of Medicine, Fred Hutchinson Cancer Research Center, University of Washington, 1100 Fairview Avenue N., Seattle, WA 98109, USA.

Journal: Cancer. 2010 Feb 15;116(4 Suppl):1126-33.

Abstract Link: http://www.medifocus.com/abstracts.php?gid=HM009&ID=20127945

Go to http://www.medifocus.com/links/HM009/0212 for direct online access to the above Abstract Links.

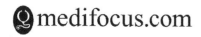

28.

Reassessing the standard of care in indolent lymphoma: a clinical update to improve clinical practice.

Author:	Rummel M
Institution:	Department for Hematology and Medical Oncology, Justus-Liebig University Hospital, Giessen, Germany.
Journal:	J Natl Compr Canc Netw. 2010 Sep;8 Suppl 6:S1-14; quiz S15.
Abstract Link:	http://www.medifocus.com/abstracts.php?gid=HM009&ID=20876549

29.

Rituximab in indolent lymphomas.

Authors:	Sousou T; Friedberg J
Institution:	James P. Wilmot Cancer Center, and Department of Medicine, University of Rochester, Rochester, NY, USA.
Journal:	Semin Hematol. 2010 Apr;47(2):133-42.
Abstract Link:	http://www.medifocus.com/abstracts.php?gid=HM009&ID=20350660

30.

Plerixafor: A chemokine receptor-4 antagonist for mobilization of hematopoietic stem cells for transplantation after high-dose chemotherapy for non-Hodgkin's lymphoma or multiple myeloma.

Authors:	Steinberg M; Silva M
Institution:	Department of Pharmacy Practice, Massachusetts College of Pharmacy and Health Sciences, Worcester, Massachusetts 01608, USA. michael.steinberg@mcphs.edu
Journal:	Clin Ther. 2010 May;32(5):821-43.
Abstract Link:	http://www.medifocus.com/abstracts.php?gid=HM009&ID=20685493

Go to http://www.medifocus.com/links/HM009/0212 for direct online access to the above Abstract Links.

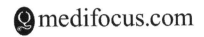
31.

Bendamustine in chronic lymphocytic leukemia and non-Hodgkin's lymphoma.

Authors:	Ujjani C; Cheson BD
Institution:	Georgetown University Hospital, Lombardi Comprehensive Cancer Center, 3800 Reservoir RD, NW, Washington, DC 20007, USA.
Journal:	Expert Rev Anticancer Ther. 2010 Sep;10(9):1353-65.
Abstract Link:	http://www.medifocus.com/abstracts.php?gid=HM009&ID=20836669

32.

Investigational histone deacetylase inhibitors for non-Hodgkin lymphomas.

Author:	Watanabe T
Institution:	National Cancer Center Hospital, Hematology Division, 5-1-1, Tsukiji, Chuo-ku, Tokyo 104-0045, Japan. takawata@ncc.go.jp
Journal:	Expert Opin Investig Drugs. 2010 Sep;19(9):1113-27.
Abstract Link:	http://www.medifocus.com/abstracts.php?gid=HM009&ID=20649502

33.

Management of non-Hodgkin lymphomas arising at extranodal sites.

Authors:	Zucca E; Gregorini A; Cavalli F
Institution:	Research Division, Oncology Institute of Southern Switzerland, Ospedale San Giovanni, Bellinzona. ielsg@ticino.com
Journal:	Ther Umsch. 2010 Oct;67(10):517-25.
Abstract Link:	http://www.medifocus.com/abstracts.php?gid=HM009&ID=20886458

Go to http://www.medifocus.com/links/HM009/0212 for direct online access to the above Abstract Links.

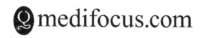

34.

Rituximab in high-grade lymphoma.

Authors:	Zwick C; Murawski N; Pfreundschuh M
Institution:	Innere Medizin I, Saarland University Medical School, Homburg, Germany.
Journal:	Semin Hematol. 2010 Apr;47(2):148-55.
Abstract Link:	http://www.medifocus.com/abstracts.php?gid=HM009&ID=20350662

35.

Management of immunocompetent patients with primary central nervous system lymphoma.

Authors:	Chimienti E; Spina M; Vaccher E; Tirelli U
Institution:	Division of Medical Oncology, National Cancer Institute, Aviano, Italy.
Journal:	Clin Lymphoma Myeloma. 2009 Oct;9(5):353-64.
Abstract Link:	http://www.medifocus.com/abstracts.php?gid=HM009&ID=19858054

36.

Prognostic factors in low-grade non-Hodgkin lymphomas.

Authors:	Federico M; Molica S; Bellei M; Luminari S
Institution:	Dipartimento di Oncologia ed Ematologia, Universita di Modena e Reggio Emilia, Centro Oncologico Modenese, Via del Pozzo, 71 41100, Modena, Italy. federico@unimore.it
Journal:	Curr Hematol Malig Rep. 2009 Oct;4(4):202-10.
Abstract Link:	http://www.medifocus.com/abstracts.php?gid=HM009&ID=20425409

Go to http://www.medifocus.com/links/HM009/0212 for direct online access to the above Abstract Links.

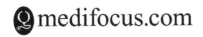

37.

Adolescent non-Hodgkin lymphoma and Hodgkin lymphoma: state of the science.

Authors:	Hochberg J; Waxman IM; Kelly KM; Morris E; Cairo MS
Institution:	Department of Pediatrics, Columbia University, New York, NY 10032, USA.
Journal:	Br J Haematol. 2009 Jan;144(1):24-40.
Abstract Link:	http://www.medifocus.com/abstracts.php?gid=HM009&ID=19087093

38.

Good things come in small packages: low-dose radiation as palliation for indolent non-Hodgkin lymphomas.

Authors:	Martin NE; Ng AK
Institution:	Harvard Radiation Oncology Program, Brigham and Women's Hospital/Dana-Farber Cancer Institute, Boston, MA 02115, USA.
Journal:	Leuk Lymphoma. 2009 Nov;50(11):1765-72.
Abstract Link:	http://www.medifocus.com/abstracts.php?gid=HM009&ID=19883306

39.

Recent developments in the treatment of aggressive non-Hodgkin lymphoma.

Authors:	Michallet AS; Coiffier B
Institution:	Hematologie, CH Lyon-Sud, 69495 Pierre-Benite, France. Anne-sophie.michallet@chu-lyon.fr
Journal:	Blood Rev. 2009 Jan;23(1):11-23. Epub 2008 Jul 11.
Abstract Link:	http://www.medifocus.com/abstracts.php?gid=HM009&ID=18620786

Go to http://www.medifocus.com/links/HM009/0212 for direct online access to the above Abstract Links.

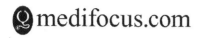

40.

Therapeutic challenges in primary CNS lymphoma.

Authors: Morris PG; Abrey LE
Institution: Department of Medicine, Memorial Sloan-Kettering Cancer Center,
                   New York, NY 10065, USA.
Journal: Lancet Neurol. 2009 Jun;8(6):581-92.
Abstract Link: http://www.medifocus.com/abstracts.php?gid=HM009&ID=19446277

41.

Radiolabeled immunotherapy in non-Hodgkin's lymphoma treatment: the next step.

Authors: Otte A; van de Wiele C; Dierckx RA
Institution: Clinical Trials Center, University Medical Center, Elsasser Str. 2,
                   D-79110 Freiburg, Germany. andreas.otte@uniklinik-freiburg.de
Journal: Nucl Med Commun. 2009 Jan;30(1):5-15.
Abstract Link: http://www.medifocus.com/abstracts.php?gid=HM009&ID=19020470

42.

Understanding the concept of uncertainty in patients with indolent lymphoma.

Author: Elphee EE
Institution: Malignant Hematology and Lymphoma Disease Site Group, Cancer
                   Care Manitoba, Canada. erin.elphee@cancercare.mb.ca
Journal: Oncol Nurs Forum. 2008 May;35(3):449-54.
Abstract Link: http://www.medifocus.com/abstracts.php?gid=HM009&ID=18467294

Go to http://www.medifocus.com/links/HM009/0212 for direct online access to the above Abstract Links.

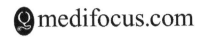

43.

Hodgkin and non-Hodgkin lymphomas during pregnancy.

Authors: Froesch P; Belisario-Filho V; Zucca E
Institution: IOSI, Oncology Institute of Southern Switzerland, Bellinzona.
Journal: Recent Results Cancer Res. 2008;178:111-21.
Abstract Link: **ABSTRACT NOT AVAILABLE**

44.

Ocrelizumab, a humanized monoclonal antibody against CD20 for inflammatory disorders and B-cell malignancies.

Author: Hutas G
Institution: Semmelweis University, Department of Rheumatology, Polyclinic of the Hospitaller Brothers of St John of God, Budapest, Hungary. gaborhutas@gmail.com
Journal: Curr Opin Investig Drugs. 2008 Nov;9(11):1206-15.
Abstract Link: http://www.medifocus.com/abstracts.php?gid=HM009&ID=18951300

45.

Oral non-Hodgkin's lymphoma: review of the literature and World Health Organization classification with reference to 40 cases.

Authors: Kemp S; Gallagher G; Kabani S; Noonan V; O'Hara C
Institution: Department of Oral and Maxillofacial Pathology, Boston University School of Dental Medicine, Boston, MA 02118, USA. skemp@bu.edu
Journal: Oral Surg Oral Med Oral Pathol Oral Radiol Endod. 2008 Feb;105(2):194-201. Epub 2007 Jun 29.
Abstract Link: http://www.medifocus.com/abstracts.php?gid=HM009&ID=17604660

Go to http://www.medifocus.com/links/HM009/0212 for direct online access to the above Abstract Links.

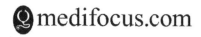

46.

Richter syndrome: a review of clinical, ocular, neurological and other manifestations.

Authors: Omoti CE; Omoti AE
Institution: Department of Haematology, University of Benin Teaching Hospital,
                     Benin City, Nigeria. ediomoti@yahoo.com
Journal: Br J Haematol. 2008 Sep;142(5):709-16. Epub 2008 May 19.
Abstract Link: http://www.medifocus.com/abstracts.php?gid=HM009&ID=18492119

47.

18F-FDG PET for posttherapy assessment of Hodgkin's disease and aggressive Non-Hodgkin's lymphoma: a systematic review.

Authors: Terasawa T; Nihashi T; Hotta T; Nagai H
Institution: Clinical Research Center for Blood Diseases, National Hospital
                     Organization Nagoya Medical Center, Nagoya, Japan.
                     tterasawa@tufts-nemc.org
Journal: J Nucl Med. 2008 Jan;49(1):13-21. Epub 2007 Dec 12.
Abstract Link: http://www.medifocus.com/abstracts.php?gid=HM009&ID=18077527

48.

Sun exposure and non-Hodgkin lymphoma.

Authors: Armstrong BK; Kricker A
Institution: Sydney Cancer Centre, Royal Prince Alfred Hospital, Missenden Road,
                     Camperdown 2050, Sydney, New South Wales, Australia.
                     brucea@health.usyd.edu.au
Journal: Cancer Epidemiol Biomarkers Prev. 2007 Mar;16(3):396-400. Epub
                     2007 Mar 2.
Abstract Link: http://www.medifocus.com/abstracts.php?gid=HM009&ID=17337644

Go to http://www.medifocus.com/links/HM009/0212 for direct online access to the above Abstract Links.

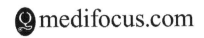

49.

Polychlorinated biphenyls and non-Hodgkin lymphoma.

Authors: Engel LS; Lan Q; Rothman N

Institution: Department of Epidemiology, Memorial Sloan-Kettering Cancer Center, Epidemiology Service, 307 E. 63rd St., 3rd Floor, New York, NY 10021, USA. engell@mskcc.org

Journal: Cancer Epidemiol Biomarkers Prev. 2007 Mar;16(3):373-6. Epub 2007 Mar 2.

Abstract Link: http://www.medifocus.com/abstracts.php?gid=HM009&ID=17337641

50.

Infectious agents as causes of non-Hodgkin lymphoma.

Author: Engels EA

Institution: Division of Cancer Epidemiology and Genetics, National Cancer Institute, NIH, Department of Health and Human Services, 6120 Executive Boulevard, EPS 7076, Rockville, MD 20852, USA. engelse@exchange.nih.gov

Journal: Cancer Epidemiol Biomarkers Prev. 2007 Mar;16(3):401-4. Epub 2007 Mar 2.

Abstract Link: http://www.medifocus.com/abstracts.php?gid=HM009&ID=17337646

51.

Primary gastric lymphoma pathogenesis and treatment: what has changed over the past 10 years?

Authors: Ferrucci PF; Zucca E

Institution: Department of Haematoncology, European Institute of Oncology (IEO), Milan, Italy. pier.ferrucci@ieo.it

Journal: Br J Haematol. 2007 Feb;136(4):521-38. Epub 2006 Dec 8.

Abstract Link: http://www.medifocus.com/abstracts.php?gid=HM009&ID=17156403

Go to http://www.medifocus.com/links/HM009/0212 for direct online access to the above Abstract Links.

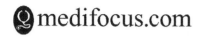

52.

Primary CNS lymphoma.

Authors:	Gerstner E; Batchelor T
Institution:	Massachusetts General Hospital and Harvard Medical School, Department of Neurology, Boston, MA 02114, USA. egerstner@partners.org
Journal:	Expert Rev Anticancer Ther. 2007 May;7(5):689-700.
Abstract Link:	http://www.medifocus.com/abstracts.php?gid=HM009&ID=17492932

53.

Altered immunity as a risk factor for non-Hodgkin lymphoma.

Authors:	Grulich AE; Vajdic CM; Cozen W
Institution:	National Centre in HIV Epidemiology and Clinical Research, Level 2, 376 Victoria Street, Darlinghurst, NSW 2010, Australia. agrulich@nchecr.unsw.edu.au
Journal:	Cancer Epidemiol Biomarkers Prev. 2007 Mar;16(3):405-8. Epub 2007 Mar 2.
Abstract Link:	http://www.medifocus.com/abstracts.php?gid=HM009&ID=17337643

54.

Management of peripheral T-cell non-Hodgkin's lymphoma.

Author:	Horwitz SM
Institution:	Memorial Sloan Kettering Cancer Center, New York, New York 10021, USA. horwitzs@mskcc.org
Journal:	Curr Opin Oncol. 2007 Sep;19(5):438-43.
Abstract Link:	http://www.medifocus.com/abstracts.php?gid=HM009&ID=17762567

Go to http://www.medifocus.com/links/HM009/0212 for direct online access to the above Abstract Links.

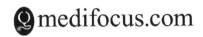
55.

Targeted therapies for non-Hodgkin lymphoma: rationally designed combinations.

Authors:	Martin P; Leonard JP
Institution:	Center for Lymphoma and Myeloma, Division of Hematology and Medical Oncology, Weill Medical College of Cornell University and New York Presbyterian Hospital, New York, NY 10021, USA.
Journal:	Clin Lymphoma Myeloma. 2007 Aug;7 Suppl 5:S192-8.
Abstract Link:	http://www.medifocus.com/abstracts.php?gid=HM009&ID=17877844

56.

Modern management of non-Hodgkin lymphoma in HIV-infected patients.

Authors:	Mounier N; Spina M; Gisselbrecht C
Institution:	Groupe d'Etude des Lymphomes de l'Adulte, GELA, 1 av C Vellefaux, Paris, France. mounier.n@chu-nice.fr
Journal:	Br J Haematol. 2007 Mar;136(5):685-98. Epub 2006 Dec 1.
Abstract Link:	http://www.medifocus.com/abstracts.php?gid=HM009&ID=17229246

57.

Obesity, diet and risk of non-Hodgkin lymphoma.

Author:	Skibola CF
Institution:	Division of Environmental Health Sciences, School of Public Health, 140 Earl Warren Hall, University of California, Berkeley, CA 94720-7360, USA. chrisfs@berkeley.edu
Journal:	Cancer Epidemiol Biomarkers Prev. 2007 Mar;16(3):392-5. Epub 2007 Mar 2.
Abstract Link:	http://www.medifocus.com/abstracts.php?gid=HM009&ID=17337642

Go to http://www.medifocus.com/links/HM009/0212 for direct online access to the above Abstract Links.

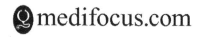

58.

Benzene exposure and risk of non-Hodgkin lymphoma.

Authors: Smith MT; Jones RM; Smith AH

Institution: Center for Occupational and Environmental Health, School of Public Health, 216 Earl Warren Hall, University of California, Berkeley, CA 94720-7360, USA. martynts@berkeley.edu

Journal: Cancer Epidemiol Biomarkers Prev. 2007 Mar;16(3):385-91. Epub 2007 Mar 2.

Abstract Link: http://www.medifocus.com/abstracts.php?gid=HM009&ID=17337645

59.

Low-grade non-hodgkin lymphomas.

Authors: Tsang RW; Gospodarowicz MK

Institution: Department of Radiation Oncology, University of Toronto, Princess Margaret Hospital, Toronto, Ontario, Canada. Richard.tsang@rmp.uhn.on.ca

Journal: Semin Radiat Oncol. 2007 Jul;17(3):198-205.

Abstract Link: http://www.medifocus.com/abstracts.php?gid=HM009&ID=17591567

60.

Incidence, risk factors, and pathogenesis of second malignancies in patients with non-Hodgkin lymphoma.

Authors: Tward J; Glenn M; Pulsipher M; Barnette P; Gaffney D

Institution: Huntsman Cancer Hospital, University of Utah, UT 84112-5560, USA. Jonathan.Tward@hci.utah.edu

Journal: Leuk Lymphoma. 2007 Aug;48(8):1482-95.

Abstract Link: http://www.medifocus.com/abstracts.php?gid=HM009&ID=17701578

Go to http://www.medifocus.com/links/HM009/0212 for direct online access to the above Abstract Links.

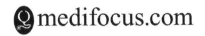

General Interest Articles

61.

Maternal smoking during pregnancy and childhood lymphoma: a meta-analysis.

Authors:	Antonopoulos CN; Sergentanis TN; Papadopoulou C; Andrie E; Dessypris N; Panagopoulou P; Polychronopoulou S; Pourtsidis A; Athanasiadou-Piperopoulou F; Kalmanti M; Sidi V; Moschovi M; Petridou ET
Institution:	Department of Hygiene, Epidemiology and Medical Statistics, Athens University Medical School, Athens, Greece.
Journal:	Int J Cancer. 2011 Dec 1;129(11):2694-703. doi: 10.1002/ijc.25929. Epub 2011 Mar 25.
Abstract Link:	http://www.medifocus.com/abstracts.php?gid=HM009&ID=21225624

62.

Sexual well-being among survivors of non-Hodgkin lymphoma.

Authors:	Beckjord EB; Arora NK; Bellizzi K; Hamilton AS; Rowland JH
Institution:	Department of Psychiatry, University of Pittsburgh, Pennsylvania, USA. beckjorde@upmc.edu
Journal:	Oncol Nurs Forum. 2011 Sep;38(5):E351-9.
Abstract Link:	http://www.medifocus.com/abstracts.php?gid=HM009&ID=21875831

63.

Non-Hodgkin's lymphoma in adolescents: experiences in 378 adolescent NHL patients treated according to pediatric NHL-BFM protocols.

Authors:	Burkhardt B; Oschlies I; Klapper W; Zimmermann M; Woessmann W; Meinhardt A; Landmann E; Attarbaschi A; Niggli F; Schrappe M; Reiter A
Institution:	NHL-BFM Study Center, Department of Pediatric Hematology and Oncology, Justus Liebig University, Giessen, Germany. birgit.burkhardt@paediat.med.uni-giessen.de
Journal:	Leukemia. 2011 Jan;25(1):153-60. Epub 2010 Oct 29.
Abstract Link:	http://www.medifocus.com/abstracts.php?gid=HM009&ID=21030984

Go to http://www.medifocus.com/links/HM009/0212 for direct online access to the above Abstract Links.

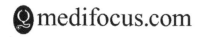

64.

Extranodal dissemination of non-Hodgkin lymphoma requires CD47 and is inhibited by anti-CD47 antibody therapy.

Authors:	Chao MP; Tang C; Pachynski RK; Chin R; Majeti R; Weissman IL
Institution:	Institute for Stem Cell Biology and Regenerative Medicine, Stanford Cancer Center, and Ludwig Center at Stanford, Stanford, CA, USA. mpchao@stanford.edu
Journal:	Blood. 2011 Nov 3;118(18):4890-901. Epub 2011 Aug 9.
Abstract Link:	http://www.medifocus.com/abstracts.php?gid=HM009&ID=21828138

65.

Dietary intake of fruit and vegetables and risk of non-Hodgkin lymphoma.

Authors:	Chiu BC; Kwon S; Evens AM; Surawicz T; Smith SM; Weisenburger DD
Institution:	Department of Health Studies, University of Chicago, 5841 South Maryland Avenue, MC 2007, Chicago, IL 60637, USA. bchiu@uchicago.edu
Journal:	Cancer Causes Control. 2011 Aug;22(8):1183-95. Epub 2011 Jun 22.
Abstract Link:	http://www.medifocus.com/abstracts.php?gid=HM009&ID=21695384

66.

The role of predictor factors in patients with non Hodgkin lymphoma in relation to the applied therapy.

Authors:	Hasic S; Arnautovic A; Jovic S; Halilbasic A; Mazalovic E
Institution:	Clinic for Oncology, Hematology and Radiotherapy, Department of Hematology, University Clinical Center Tuzla, Tuzla, Bosnia and Herzegovina. samira.hasic@ukc.ba
Journal:	Med Arh. 2011;65(2):73-7.
Abstract Link:	http://www.medifocus.com/abstracts.php?gid=HM009&ID=21585177

Go to http://www.medifocus.com/links/HM009/0212 for direct online access to the above Abstract Links.

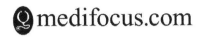

67.

Cigarette smoking, passive smoking, and non-Hodgkin lymphoma risk: evidence from the California Teachers Study.

Authors:	Lu Y; Wang SS; Reynolds P; Chang ET; Ma H; Sullivan-Halley J; Clarke CA; Bernstein L
Institution:	Department of Population Sciences, Beckman Research Institute, City of Hope, 1500 East Duarte Road, Duarte, CA 91010, USA. yalu@coh.org
Journal:	Am J Epidemiol. 2011 Sep 1;174(5):563-73. Epub 2011 Jul 18.
Abstract Link:	http://www.medifocus.com/abstracts.php?gid=HM009&ID=21768403

68.

Survival among patients with primary central nervous system lymphoma, 1973-2004.

Authors:	Norden AD; Drappatz J; Wen PY; Claus EB
Institution:	Center for Neuro-Oncology, Dana-Farber/Brigham and Women's Cancer Center, 44 Binney St, Boston, MA 02115, USA. anorden@partners.org
Journal:	J Neurooncol. 2011 Feb;101(3):487-93. Epub 2010 Jun 17.
Abstract Link:	http://www.medifocus.com/abstracts.php?gid=HM009&ID=20556477

69.

Risk for second malignancies in non-Hodgkin's lymphoma survivors: a meta-analysis.

Authors:	Pirani M; Marcheselli R; Marcheselli L; Bari A; Federico M; Sacchi S
Institution:	Department of Oncology and Hematology, University of Modena and Reggio Emilia, Modena, Italy.
Journal:	Ann Oncol. 2011 Aug;22(8):1845-58. Epub 2011 Feb 10.
Abstract Link:	http://www.medifocus.com/abstracts.php?gid=HM009&ID=21310758

Go to http://www.medifocus.com/links/HM009/0212 for direct online access to the above Abstract Links.

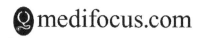 medifocus.com

---

70.

Post-traumatic stress symptoms in long-term non-Hodgkin's lymphoma survivors: does time heal?

Authors:	Smith SK; Zimmerman S; Williams CS; Benecha H; Abernethy AP; Mayer DK; Edwards LJ; Ganz PA
Institution:	Duke University Medical Center, DUMC 2732, Durham, NC 27710, USA. sophia.smith@duke.edu
Journal:	J Clin Oncol. 2011 Dec 1;29(34):4526-33. Epub 2011 Oct 11.
Abstract Link:	http://www.medifocus.com/abstracts.php?gid=HM009&ID=21990412

71.

Improving relative survival, but large remaining differences in survival for non-Hodgkin's lymphoma across Europe and the United States from 1990 to 2004.

Authors:	van de Schans SA; Gondos A; van Spronsen DJ; Rachtan J; Holleczek B; Zanetti R; Coebergh JW; Janssen-Heijnen ML; Brenner H
Institution:	Comprehensive Cancer Centre South, Eindhoven Cancer Registry, Eindhoven, The Netherlands. research@ikz.nl
Journal:	J Clin Oncol. 2011 Jan 10;29(2):192-9. Epub 2010 Nov 29.
Abstract Link:	http://www.medifocus.com/abstracts.php?gid=HM009&ID=21115853

72.

Allogeneic natural killer cells for refractory lymphoma.

Authors:	Bachanova V; Burns LJ; McKenna DH; Curtsinger J; Panoskaltsis-Mortari A; Lindgren BR; Cooley S; Weisdorf D; Miller JS
Institution:	Blood and Marrow, Transplant Program, University of Minnesota, Minneapolis, MN 55455, USA. bach0173@umn.edu
Journal:	Cancer Immunol Immunother. 2010 Nov;59(11):1739-44. Epub 2010 Aug 3.
Abstract Link:	http://www.medifocus.com/abstracts.php?gid=HM009&ID=20680271

Go to http://www.medifocus.com/links/HM009/0212 for direct online access to the above Abstract Links.

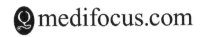

73.

Non-Hodgkin's lymphoma in the elderly.

Authors: Caimi PF; Barr PM; Berger NA; Lazarus HM

Institution: Department of Medicine, Case Comprehensive Cancer Center, University Hospitals Case Medical Center, Case Western Reserve University, Cleveland, Ohio 44106, USA.

Journal: Drugs Aging. 2010 Mar 1;27(3):211-38. doi: 10.2165/11531550-000000000-00000.

Abstract Link: http://www.medifocus.com/abstracts.php?gid=HM009&ID=20210368

74.

Characteristics and outcomes of elderly patients with primary central nervous system lymphoma: the Memorial Sloan-Kettering Cancer Center experience.

Authors: Ney DE; Reiner AS; Panageas KS; Brown HS; DeAngelis LM; Abrey LE

Institution: Department of Neurology, Memorial Sloan-Kettering Cancer Center, New York, New York 10065, USA.

Journal: Cancer. 2010 Oct 1;116(19):4605-12.

Abstract Link: http://www.medifocus.com/abstracts.php?gid=HM009&ID=20572045

75.

Primary gastrointestinal non-Hodgkin lymphoma in adults: clinicopathologic and survival characteristics.

Authors: Radic-Kristo D; Planinc-Peraica A; Ostojic S; Vrhovac R; Kardum-Skelin I; Jaksic B

Institution: Department of Medicine, "Merkur" University Hospital, Zagreb, Croatia. delfaradic@kb.merkur.com

Journal: Coll Antropol. 2010 Jun;34(2):413-7.

Abstract Link: http://www.medifocus.com/abstracts.php?gid=HM009&ID=20698111

Go to http://www.medifocus.com/links/HM009/0212 for direct online access to the above Abstract Links.

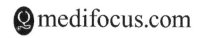

76.

NCCN Clinical Practice Guidelines in Oncology: non-Hodgkin's lymphomas.

Authors:	Zelenetz AD; Abramson JS; Advani RH; Andreadis CB; Byrd JC; Czuczman MS; Fayad L; Forero A; Glenn MJ; Gockerman JP; Gordon LI; Harris NL; Hoppe RT; Horwitz SM; Kaminski MS; Kim YH; Lacasce AS; Mughal TI; Nademanee A; Porcu P; Press O; Prosnitz L; Reddy N; Smith MR; Sokol L; Swinnen L; Vose JM; Wierda WG; Yahalom J; Yunus F
Journal:	J Natl Compr Canc Netw. 2010 Mar;8(3):288-334.
Abstract Link:	**ABSTRACT NOT AVAILABLE**

77.

Physical activity and quality of life in adult survivors of non-Hodgkin's lymphoma.

Authors:	Bellizzi KM; Rowland JH; Arora NK; Hamilton AS; Miller MF; Aziz NM
Institution:	Department of Human Development and Family Studies, University of Connecticut, 348 Mansfield Rd, Unit 2058, Storrs, CT 06269, USA. Keith.M.Bellizzi@Uconn.edu
Journal:	J Clin Oncol. 2009 Feb 20;27(6):960-6. Epub 2009 Jan 12.
Abstract Link:	http://www.medifocus.com/abstracts.php?gid=HM009&ID=19139438

78.

Accelerated R-COP: a pilot study for the treatment of advanced low grade lymphomas that has a high complete response rate.

Authors:	Levitt MJ; Gharibo M; Strair R; Schaar D; Rubin A; Bertino JR
Institution:	Department of Medicine, University of Medicine and Dentistry, Robert Wood Johnson Medical School, and The Cancer Institute of New Jersey, New Brusnwick, NJ 08901, USA.
Journal:	J Chemother. 2009 Aug;21(4):434-8.
Abstract Link:	http://www.medifocus.com/abstracts.php?gid=HM009&ID=19622463

Go to http://www.medifocus.com/links/HM009/0212 for direct online access to the above Abstract Links.

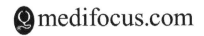 medifocus.com

---

79.

Long-term survival of patients diagnosed with non-Hodgkin lymphoma after a previous malignancy.

Authors:	Pulte D; Gondos A; Brenner H
Institution:	Division of Clinical Epidemiology and Aging Research, German Cancer Research Center, Heidelberg, Germany.
Journal:	Leuk Lymphoma. 2009 Feb;50(2):179-86.
Abstract Link:	http://www.medifocus.com/abstracts.php?gid=HM009&ID=19197735

80.

Health status and quality of life among non-Hodgkin lymphoma survivors.

Authors:	Smith SK; Zimmerman S; Williams CS; Zebrack BJ
Institution:	Sheps Center for Health Services Research, University of North Carolina, Chapel Hill, NC, USA. sophia_smith@unc.edu
Journal:	Cancer. 2009 Jul 15;115(14):3312-23.
Abstract Link:	http://www.medifocus.com/abstracts.php?gid=HM009&ID=19452546

81.

Management of unfit patients with unfavourable non-Hodgkin's lymphomas.

Authors:	Soubeyran P; Mertens C; Bellera C; Mathoulin-Pelissier S; Rainfray M
Institution:	Medical Oncology Department, Institut Bergonie, 33076 Bordeaux Cedex, France. Soubeyran_p@bergonie.org
Journal:	Cancer Treat Rev. 2009 Oct;35(6):528-32. Epub 2009 Sep 16.
Abstract Link:	http://www.medifocus.com/abstracts.php?gid=HM009&ID=19762154

Go to http://www.medifocus.com/links/HM009/0212 for direct online access to the above Abstract Links.

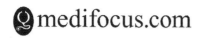

82.

Population-based analysis of incidence and outcome of transformed non-Hodgkin's lymphoma.

Authors:	Al-Tourah AJ; Gill KK; Chhanabhai M; Hoskins PJ; Klasa RJ; Savage KJ; Sehn LH; Shenkier TN; Gascoyne RD; Connors JM
Institution:	Division of Medical Oncology, Fraser Valley and Vancouver Cancer Centers and the Department of Pathology and Biostatistics, British Columbia Cancer Agency and the University of British Columbia, Vancouver, BC, Canada. aaltoura@bccancer.bc.ca
Journal:	J Clin Oncol. 2008 Nov 10;26(32):5165-9. Epub 2008 Oct 6.
Abstract Link:	http://www.medifocus.com/abstracts.php?gid=HM009&ID=18838711

83.

Survival patterns among lymphoma patients with a family history of lymphoma.

Authors:	Anderson LA; Pfeiffer RM; Rapkin JS; Gridley G; Mellemkjaer L; Hemminki K; Bjorkholm M; Caporaso NE; Landgren O
Institution:	Viral Epidemiology Branch, Division of Cancer Epidemiology and Genetics, National Cancer Institute, NIH, Bethesda, MD 20892, USA. l.anderson@qub.ac.uk
Journal:	J Clin Oncol. 2008 Oct 20;26(30):4958-65. Epub 2008 Jul 7.
Abstract Link:	http://www.medifocus.com/abstracts.php?gid=HM009&ID=18606984

84.

Incidence and mortality from non-Hodgkin lymphoma in Europe: the end of an epidemic?

Authors:	Bosetti C; Levi F; Ferlay J; Lucchini F; Negri E; La Vecchia C
Institution:	Istituto di Ricerche Farmacologiche Mario Negri, Milan, Italy. bosetti@marionegri.it
Journal:	Int J Cancer. 2008 Oct 15;123(8):1917-23.
Abstract Link:	http://www.medifocus.com/abstracts.php?gid=HM009&ID=18688859

Go to http://www.medifocus.com/links/HM009/0212 for direct online access to the above Abstract Links.

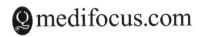

85.

Malignant non-Hodgkin's lymphoma (NHL) of the jaws: a review of 16 cases.

Authors:	Djavanmardi L; Oprean N; Alantar A; Bousetta K; Princ G
Institution:	Tunisia private practice.
Journal:	J Craniomaxillofac Surg. 2008 Oct;36(7):410-4. Epub 2008 Jun 17.
Abstract Link:	http://www.medifocus.com/abstracts.php?gid=HM009&ID=18562205

86.

Primary central nervous system lymphoma: the role of consolidation treatment after a complete response to high-dose methotrexate-based chemotherapy.

Authors:	Ekenel M; Iwamoto FM; Ben-Porat LS; Panageas KS; Yahalom J; DeAngelis LM; Abrey LE
Institution:	Department of Neurology, Memorial Sloan-Kettering Cancer Center, New York, New York 10065, USA.
Journal:	Cancer. 2008 Sep 1;113(5):1025-31.
Abstract Link:	http://www.medifocus.com/abstracts.php?gid=HM009&ID=18618509

87.

Secondary malignancies after therapy of indolent non-Hodgkin's lymphoma.

Author:	Friedberg JW
Journal:	Haematologica. 2008 Mar;93(3):336-8.
Abstract Link:	**ABSTRACT NOT AVAILABLE**

Go to http://www.medifocus.com/links/HM009/0212 for direct online access to the above Abstract Links.

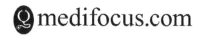

88.

Non-Hodgkin lymphoma in women: reproductive factors and exogenous hormone use.

Authors: Lee JS; Bracci PM; Holly EA
Institution: Division of Endocrinology, Clinical Nutrition, and Vascular Medicine, Department of Internal Medicine, University of California Davis, Sacramento, CA, USA.
Journal: Am J Epidemiol. 2008 Aug 1;168(3):278-88. Epub 2008 Jun 10.
Abstract Link: http://www.medifocus.com/abstracts.php?gid=HM009&ID=18550561

89.

Interstitial pneumonitis during rituximab-containing chemotherapy for non-Hodgkin lymphoma.

Authors: Liu X; Hong XN; Gu YJ; Wang BY; Luo ZG; Cao J
Institution: Department of Medical Oncology, Fudan University Cancer Hospital, Shanghai, China.
Journal: Leuk Lymphoma. 2008 Sep;49(9):1778-83.
Abstract Link: http://www.medifocus.com/abstracts.php?gid=HM009&ID=18798110

90.

Cancer risks among relatives of children with Hodgkin and non-Hodgkin lymphoma.

Authors: Pang D; Alston RD; Eden TO; Birch JM
Institution: University of Manchester and Cancer Research UK, Paediatric and Familial Cancer Research Group, Royal Manchester Children's Hospital, Manchester, United Kingdom. dong.pang@manchester.ac.uk
Journal: Int J Cancer. 2008 Sep 15;123(6):1407-10.
Abstract Link: http://www.medifocus.com/abstracts.php?gid=HM009&ID=18561317

Go to http://www.medifocus.com/links/HM009/0212 for direct online access to the above Abstract Links.

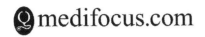

91.

Ongoing improvement in outcomes for patients diagnosed as having Non-Hodgkin lymphoma from the 1990s to the early 21st century.

Authors:	Pulte D; Gondos A; Brenner H
Institution:	Division of Clinical Epidemiology & Aging Research, German Cancer Research Center, Bergheimer Strasse 20, D-69115 Heidelberg, Germany.

Journal:	Arch Intern Med. 2008 Mar 10;168(5):469-76.
Abstract Link:	http://www.medifocus.com/abstracts.php?gid=HM009&ID=18332290

92.

Secondary malignancies after treatment for indolent non-Hodgkin's lymphoma: a 16-year follow-up study.

Authors:	Sacchi S; Marcheselli L; Bari A; Marcheselli R; Pozzi S; Luminari S; Lombardo M; Buda G; Lazzaro A; Gobbi PG; Stelitano C; Morabito F; Quarta G; Brugiatelli M
Institution:	Dipartimento di Oncologia ed Ematologia, Universita di Modena Centro Oncologico Modenese Policlinico, 41100 Modena, Italy. ssacchi@unimo.it

Journal:	Haematologica. 2008 Mar;93(3):398-404. Epub 2008 Feb 11.
Abstract Link:	http://www.medifocus.com/abstracts.php?gid=HM009&ID=18268277

93.

Non-Hodgkin's lymphoma in very elderly patients over 80 years. A descriptive analysis of clinical presentation and outcome.

Authors:	Thieblemont C; Grossoeuvre A; Houot R; Broussais-Guillaumont F; Salles G; Traulle C; Espinouse D; Coiffier B
Institution:	Departement d'Hematologie Clinique, Assistance Publique des Hopitaux de Paris, Hopital Saint-Louis, Institut Universitaire d'Hematologie, Paris. catherine.thieblemont@sls.aphp.fr

Journal:	Ann Oncol. 2008 Apr;19(4):774-9. Epub 2007 Dec 6.
Abstract Link:	http://www.medifocus.com/abstracts.php?gid=HM009&ID=18065404

Go to http://www.medifocus.com/links/HM009/0212 for direct online access to the above Abstract Links.

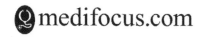

94.

Clinical significance of axillary findings in patients with lymphoma during follow-up with 18F-fluorodeoxyglucose-PET.

Authors: Tsamita CS; Golemi A; Egesta L; Castellucci P; Nanni C; Stefoni V; Grassetto G; Rubello D; Tani M; Zinzani PL; Fanti S

Institution: Department of Nuclear Medicine, Institute of Emathology, Policlinico S. Orsola-Malpighi, Bologna, Italy.

Journal: Nucl Med Commun. 2008 Aug;29(8):705-10.

Abstract Link: http://www.medifocus.com/abstracts.php?gid=HM009&ID=18753823

95.

Occupation and the risk of non-Hodgkin lymphoma.

Authors: Boffetta P; de Vocht F

Institution: Gene-Environment Epidemiology Group, IARC, 150 cours Albert-Thomas, 69008 Lyon, France. boffetta@iarc.fr

Journal: Cancer Epidemiol Biomarkers Prev. 2007 Mar;16(3):369-72.

Abstract Link: http://www.medifocus.com/abstracts.php?gid=HM009&ID=17372232

96.

Elderly patients with non-Hodgkin lymphoma who receive chemotherapy are at higher risk for osteoporosis and fractures.

Authors: Cabanillas ME; Lu H; Fang S; Du XL

Institution: Department of Leukemia, The University of Texas M.D. Anderson Cancer Center, Houston, TX, USA. mcabani@mdanderson.org

Journal: Leuk Lymphoma. 2007 Aug;48(8):1514-21.

Abstract Link: http://www.medifocus.com/abstracts.php?gid=HM009&ID=17701582

Go to http://www.medifocus.com/links/HM009/0212 for direct online access to the above Abstract Links.

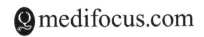

97.

The role of surgical intervention in non-Hodgkin's lymphoma of the colon and rectum.

Authors:	Cai S; Cannizzo F Jr; Bullard Dunn KM; Gibbs JF; Czuczman M; Rajput A
Institution:	Department of Surgery, The State University of New York at Buffalo, Buffalo, NY, USA.

Journal: Am J Surg. 2007 Mar;193(3):409-12; discussion 412.
Abstract Link: http://www.medifocus.com/abstracts.php?gid=HM009&ID=17320545

98.

Immunogenicity of influenza vaccination in patients with non-hodgkin lymphoma.

Authors:	Centkowski P; Brydak L; Machala M; Kalinka-Warzocha E; Blasinska-Morawiec M; Federowicz I; Walewski J; Wc E Grzyn J; Wolowiec D; Lech-Maranda E; Sawczuk-Chabin J; Bilinski P; Warzocha K
Institution:	Department of Hematology, Institute of Hematology and Transfusion Medicine, I. Gandhi Street 14, 02776, Warsaw, Poland.

Journal: J Clin Immunol. 2007 May;27(3):339-46. Epub 2007 Mar 8.
Abstract Link: http://www.medifocus.com/abstracts.php?gid=HM009&ID=17345151

99.

Revised response criteria for malignant lymphoma.

Authors:	Cheson BD; Pfistner B; Juweid ME; Gascoyne RD; Specht L; Horning SJ; Coiffier B; Fisher RI; Hagenbeek A; Zucca E; Rosen ST; Stroobants S; Lister TA; Hoppe RT; Dreyling M; Tobinai K; Vose JM; Connors JM; Federico M; Diehl V
Institution:	Division of Hematology/Oncology, Georgetown University Hospital, Washington, DC, USA. bdc4@georgetown.edu

Journal: J Clin Oncol. 2007 Feb 10;25(5):579-86. Epub 2007 Jan 22.
Abstract Link: http://www.medifocus.com/abstracts.php?gid=HM009&ID=17242396

Go to http://www.medifocus.com/links/HM009/0212 for direct online access to the above Abstract Links.

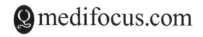

100.

Obesity and risk of non-Hodgkin lymphoma (United States).

Authors:	Chiu BC; Soni L; Gapstur SM; Fought AJ; Evens AM; Weisenburger DD
Institution:	Department of Preventive Medicine, Feinberg School of Medicine, Northwestern University, 680 North Lake Shore Drive, Suite 1102, Chicago, IL, 60611-4402, USA.
Journal:	Cancer Causes Control. 2007 May 7;.
Abstract Link:	http://www.medifocus.com/abstracts.php?gid=HM009&ID=17484069

101.

Survival from adolescent cancer.

Author:	Desandes E
Institution:	French National Registry of Childhood Solid Tumours, Universite Henri Poincare Nancy 1, Faculte de Medecine, 9, Avenue de la Foret de Haye, BP 184, 54505 Vandoeuvre-les-Nancy cedex, France.
Journal:	Cancer Treat Rev. 2007 Mar 28;.
Abstract Link:	http://www.medifocus.com/abstracts.php?gid=HM009&ID=17398011

102.

Environmental and behavioral factors and the risk of non-Hodgkin lymphoma.

Authors:	Hartge P; Smith MT
Institution:	National Cancer Institute, NIH, Department of Health and Human Services, Rockville, MD 20892, USA. hartge@nih.gov
Journal:	Cancer Epidemiol Biomarkers Prev. 2007 Mar;16(3):367-8. Epub 2007 Mar 7.
Abstract Link:	**ABSTRACT NOT AVAILABLE**

Go to http://www.medifocus.com/links/HM009/0212 for direct online access to the above Abstract Links.

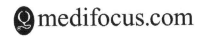

103.

Clinical characteristics and treatment results of pediatric B-cell non-Hodgkin lymphoma patients in a single center.

Authors:	Karadeniz C; Oguz A; Citak EC; Uluoglu O; Okur V; Demirci S; Okur A; Aksakal N
Institution:	Gazi University Faculty of Medicine, Department of Pediatric Oncology, Ankara, Turkey.
Journal:	Pediatr Hematol Oncol. 2007 Sep;24(6):417-30.
Abstract Link:	http://www.medifocus.com/abstracts.php?gid=HM009&ID=17710659

104.

Rheumatic manifestations of lymphoproliferative disorders.

Authors:	Kiltz U; Brandt J; Zochling J; Braun J
Institution:	Rheumazentrum Ruhrgebiet, St. Josefs-Krankenhaus, Herne, Germany. kiltz@rheumazentrum-ruhrgbiet.de
Journal:	Clin Exp Rheumatol. 2007 Jan-Feb;25(1):35-9.
Abstract Link:	http://www.medifocus.com/abstracts.php?gid=HM009&ID=17417988

105.

The role of FDG PET in the management of lymphoma: what is the evidence base?

Authors:	Kirby AM; Mikhaeel NG
Institution:	Department of Clinical Oncology, Guy's and St Thomas' NHS Trust, London, UK. annakirby@doctors.org.uk
Journal:	Nucl Med Commun. 2007 May;28(5):335-54.
Abstract Link:	http://www.medifocus.com/abstracts.php?gid=HM009&ID=17414883

Go to http://www.medifocus.com/links/HM009/0212 for direct online access to the above Abstract Links.

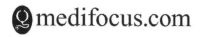
106.

Predicting the outcome in non-Hodgkin lymphoma with molecular markers.

Author:	Kwong YL
Institution:	Department of Medicine, University of Hong Kong, Hong Kong, China.
Journal:	Br J Haematol. 2007 May;137(4):273-87. Epub 2007 Apr 4.
Abstract Link:	http://www.medifocus.com/abstracts.php?gid=HM009&ID=17408399

107.

Risk of second malignant neoplasms after childhood leukemia and lymphoma: an international study.

Authors:	Maule M; Scelo G; Pastore G; Brennan P; Hemminki K; Tracey E; Sankila R; Weiderpass E; Olsen JH; McBride ML; Brewster DH; Pompe-Kirn V; Kliewer EV; Chia KS; Tonita JM; Martos C; Jonasson JG; Merletti F; Boffetta P
Institution:	Childhood Cancer Registry of Piedmont, Cancer Epidemiology Unit, CPO Piemonte, CeRMS, University of Turin, Via Santena 7, 10126, Turin, Italy. milena.maule@unito.it
Journal:	J Natl Cancer Inst. 2007 May 16;99(10):790-800.
Abstract Link:	http://www.medifocus.com/abstracts.php?gid=HM009&ID=17505074

108.

Quality of life among long-term non-Hodgkin lymphoma survivors: a population-based study.

Authors:	Mols F; Aaronson NK; Vingerhoets AJ; Coebergh JW; Vreugdenhil G; Lybeert ML; van de Poll-Franse LV
Institution:	Comprehensive Cancer Center South, Eindhoven Cancer Registry, Eindhoven, the Netherlands. f.mols@uvt.nl
Journal:	Cancer. 2007 Apr 15;109(8):1659-67.
Abstract Link:	http://www.medifocus.com/abstracts.php?gid=HM009&ID=17330853

Go to http://www.medifocus.com/links/HM009/0212 for direct online access to the above Abstract Links.

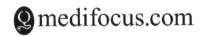

109.

Long-term pulmonary function in survivors of childhood Hodgkin disease and non-Hodgkin lymphoma.

Authors:	Oguz A; Tayfun T; Citak EC; Karadeniz C; Tatlicioglu T; Boyunaga O; Bora H
Institution:	Department of Pediatric Oncology, Gazi University Faculty of Medicine, Ankara, Turkey.
Journal:	Pediatr Blood Cancer. 2007 Apr 9;.
Abstract Link:	http://www.medifocus.com/abstracts.php?gid=HM009&ID=17420991

110.

Infectious complications of monoclonal antibodies used in cancer therapy: a systematic review of the evidence from randomized controlled trials.

Authors:	Rafailidis PI; Kakisi OK; Vardakas K; Falagas ME
Institution:	Alfa Institute of Biomedical Sciences (AIBS), Athens, Greece.
Journal:	Cancer. 2007 Apr 11;.
Abstract Link:	http://www.medifocus.com/abstracts.php?gid=HM009&ID=17429839

111.

The impact of involved field radiation therapy in the treatment of relapsed or refractory non-Hodgkin lymphoma with high-dose chemotherapy followed by hematopoietic progenitor cell transplant.

Authors:	Wendland MM; Smith DC; Boucher KM; Asch JD; Pulsipher MA; Thomson JW; Shrieve DC; Gaffney DK
Institution:	Department of Radiation Oncology, Huntsman Cancer Hospital and the University of Utah, Salt Lake City, Utah 84112, USA.
Journal:	Am J Clin Oncol. 2007 Apr;30(2):156-62.
Abstract Link:	http://www.medifocus.com/abstracts.php?gid=HM009&ID=17414465

Go to http://www.medifocus.com/links/HM009/0212 for direct online access to the above Abstract Links.

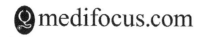

Drug Therapy Articles

112.

Poly(ADP-ribose) polymerase inhibitors combined with external beam and radioimmunotherapy to treat aggressive lymphoma.

Authors:	Li, Qiang; Liu, Yan; Zhao, Wei; Chen, Xing-Zhen; Schaefer NG; James E; Wahl RL
Institution:	Division of Nuclear Medicine, Russell H. Morgan Department of Radiology and Radiological Sciences, Sidney Kimmell Cancer Center, Johns Hopkins University School of Medicine, Baltimore, Maryland 21287-0817, USA.
Journal:	Nucl Med Commun. 2011 Nov;32(11):1046-51.
Abstract Link:	http://www.medifocus.com/abstracts.php?gid=HM009&ID=21956491

113.

Salvage therapy with gemcitabine, ifosfamide, dexamethasone, and oxaliplatin (GIDOX) for B-cell non-Hodgkin's lymphoma: a consortium for improving survival of lymphoma (CISL) trial.

Authors:	Park BB; Kim WS; Eom HS; Kim JS; Lee YY; Oh SJ; Lee DH; Suh C
Institution:	Division of Hematology/Oncology, Department of Internal Medicine, Hanyang University College of Medicine, Seoul, South Korea.
Journal:	Invest New Drugs. 2011 Feb;29(1):154-60. Epub 2009 Sep 16.
Abstract Link:	http://www.medifocus.com/abstracts.php?gid=HM009&ID=19756371

114.

Efficacy of high-dose methotrexate, ifosfamide, etoposide and dexamethasone salvage therapy for recurrent or refractory childhood malignant lymphoma.

Authors:	Sandlund JT; Pui CH; Mahmoud H; Zhou Y; Lowe E; Kaste S; Kun LE; Krasin MJ; Onciu M; Behm FG; Ribeiro RC; Razzouk BI; Howard SC; Metzger ML; Hale GA; Rencher R; Graham K; Hudson MM
Institution:	Department of Oncology, St Jude Children's Research Hospital, University of Tennessee, Memphis, TN, USA. John.Sandlund@stjude.org

Go to http://www.medifocus.com/links/HM009/0212 for direct online access to the above Abstract Links.

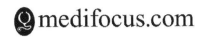

Journal:	Ann Oncol. 2011 Feb;22(2):468-71. Epub 2010 Jul 12.
Abstract Link:	http://www.medifocus.com/abstracts.php?gid=HM009&ID=20624787

115.

Standard chemotherapy is superior to high-dose chemotherapy with autologous stem cell transplantation on overall survival as the first-line therapy for patients with aggressive non-Hodgkin lymphoma: a meta-analysis.

Authors:	Wang J; Zhan P; Ouyang J; Chen B; Zhou R; Yang Y
Institution:	Department of Hematology, The Affiliated DrumTower Hospital of Nanjing University Medical School, 210008, Nanjing, People's Republic of China.
Journal:	Med Oncol. 2011 Sep;28(3):822-8. Epub 2010 Apr 6.
Abstract Link:	http://www.medifocus.com/abstracts.php?gid=HM009&ID=20373054

116.

High dose intensity doxorubicin in aggressive non-Hodgkin's lymphoma: a literature-based meta-analysis.

Authors:	Azim HA; Santoro L; Bociek RG; Gandini S; Malek RA; Azim HA Jr
Institution:	Department of Clinical Oncology, Cairo University Hospital, Cairo, Egypt.
Journal:	Ann Oncol. 2010 May;21(5):1064-71. Epub 2009 Oct 22.
Abstract Link:	http://www.medifocus.com/abstracts.php?gid=HM009&ID=19850640

117.

Anti-CD22-MCC-DM1: an antibody-drug conjugate with a stable linker for the treatment of non-Hodgkin's lymphoma.

Authors:	Polson AG; Williams M; Gray AM; Fuji RN; Poon KA; McBride J; Raab H; Januario T; Go M; Lau J; Yu SF; Du C; Fuh F; Tan C; Wu Y; Liang WC; Prabhu S; Stephan JP; Hongo JA; Dere RC; Deng R; Cullen M; de Tute R; Bennett F; Rawstron A; Jack A; Ebens A
Institution:	Research and Early Development, Genentech, South San Francisco, CA 94080, USA. polson@gene.com
Journal:	Leukemia. 2010 Sep;24(9):1566-73. Epub 2010 Jul 1.
Abstract Link:	http://www.medifocus.com/abstracts.php?gid=HM009&ID=20596033

Go to http://www.medifocus.com/links/HM009/0212 for direct online access to the above Abstract Links.

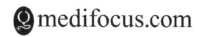

118.

Long-term results of pirarubicin versus doxorubicin in combination chemotherapy for aggressive non-Hodgkin's lymphoma: single center, 15-year experience.

Authors: Zhai L; Guo C; Cao Y; Xiao J; Fu X; Huang J; Huang H; Guan Z; Lin T

Institution: State Key Laboratory of Oncology in South China, Department of Medical Oncology, Sun Yat-Sen University Cancer Center, 651 Dong Feng Road East, 510060, Guangzhou, Guangdong, People's Republic of China.

Journal: Int J Hematol. 2010 Jan;91(1):78-86. Epub 2009 Dec 23.

Abstract Link: http://www.medifocus.com/abstracts.php?gid=HM009&ID=20033628

119.

Addition of rituximab to cyclophosphamide, doxorubicin, vincristine, and prednisolone therapy has a high risk of developing interstitial pneumonia in patients with non-Hodgkin lymphoma.

Authors: Katsuya H; Suzumiya J; Sasaki H; Ishitsuka K; Shibata T; Takamatsu Y; Tamura K

Institution: Department of Medical Oncology and Hematology, Fukuoka University Hospital, Fukuoka, Japan.

Journal: Leuk Lymphoma. 2009 Nov;50(11):1818-23.

Abstract Link: http://www.medifocus.com/abstracts.php?gid=HM009&ID=19863173

120.

Veltuzumab, an anti-CD20 mAb for the treatment of non-Hodgkin's lymphoma, chronic lymphocytic leukemia and immune thrombocytopenic purpura.

Authors: Milani C; Castillo J

Institution: Brown University Warren Alpert Medical School, The Miriam Hospital, Division of Hematology and Oncology, 164 Summit Avenue, Providence, RI 02906, USA.

Journal: Curr Opin Mol Ther. 2009 Apr;11(2):200-7.

Abstract Link: http://www.medifocus.com/abstracts.php?gid=HM009&ID=19330725

Go to http://www.medifocus.com/links/HM009/0212 for direct online access to the above Abstract Links.

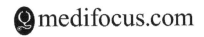

121.

Rituximab as monotherapy and in addition to reduced CHOP in children with primary immunodeficiency and non-Hodgkin lymphoma.

Authors:	Shabbat S; Aharoni J; Sarid L; Ben-Harush M; Kapelushnik J
Institution:	Department of Pediatrics, Soroka University Medical Center, Beer Sheva, Israel. shimriti@bgu.ac.il
Journal:	Pediatr Blood Cancer. 2009 May;52(5):664-6.
Abstract Link:	http://www.medifocus.com/abstracts.php?gid=HM009&ID=19142990

122.

Gemcitabine-based combination chemotherapy as salvage treatment for refractory or relapsing aggressive non-Hodgkin's lymphoma.

Authors:	Yang SH; Lin ZZ; Kuo SH; Cheng AL
Journal:	Am J Hematol. 2009 Jul;84(7):457-9.
Abstract Link:	**ABSTRACT NOT AVAILABLE**

123.

Comparison of ICE (ifosfamide-carboplatin-etoposide) versus DHAP (cytosine arabinoside-cisplatin-dexamethasone) as salvage chemotherapy in patients with relapsed or refractory lymphoma.

Authors:	Abali H; Urun Y; Oksuzoglu B; Budakoglu B; Yildirim N; Guler T; Ozet G; Zengin N
Institution:	Department of Internal Medicine, Medical Oncology Unit, Mersin University, Mersin, Turkey. habali1970@yahoo.com
Journal:	Cancer Invest. 2008 May;26(4):401-6.
Abstract Link:	http://www.medifocus.com/abstracts.php?gid=HM009&ID=18443961

Go to http://www.medifocus.com/links/HM009/0212 for direct online access to the above Abstract Links.

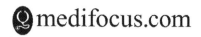

124.

Lenalidomide for the treatment of B-cell malignancies.

Authors: Chanan-Khan AA; Cheson BD
Institution: Roswell Park Cancer Institute, Buffalo, NY, USA.
                     asher.chanan-khan@roswellpark.org
Journal: J Clin Oncol. 2008 Mar 20;26(9):1544-52. Epub 2008 Feb 19.
Abstract Link: http://www.medifocus.com/abstracts.php?gid=HM009&ID=18285605

125.

Polo-like kinase 1 as a new target for non-Hodgkin's lymphoma treatment.

Authors: Liu L; Zhang M; Zou P
Institution: Department of Hematology, Union Hospital, Tongji Medical College, Huazhong University of Science and Technology, Wuhan, China.
Journal: Oncology. 2008;74(1-2):96-103. Epub 2008 Jun 12.
Abstract Link: http://www.medifocus.com/abstracts.php?gid=HM009&ID=18547964

126.

Cladribine in indolent non-Hodgkin's lymphoma.

Authors: Sigal DS; Saven A
Institution: Division of Hematology/Oncology, Scripps Clinic, 10666 N. Torrey Pines Road, M/S 217 La Jolla, CA 92037, USA.
                     sigal.darren@scrippshealth.org
Journal: Expert Rev Anticancer Ther. 2008 Apr;8(4):535-45.
Abstract Link: http://www.medifocus.com/abstracts.php?gid=HM009&ID=18402520

Go to http://www.medifocus.com/links/HM009/0212 for direct online access to the above Abstract Links.

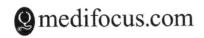
127.

Rituximab in lymphoma: a systematic review and consensus practice guideline from Cancer Care Ontario.

Authors: Cheung MC; Haynes AE; Meyer RM; Stevens A; Imrie KR

Institution: Cancer Care Ontario Program in Evidence-Based Care, McMaster University, Hamilton, Ont., Canada L8S 4L8. matthew.cheung@utoronto.ca <matthew.cheung@utoronto.ca>

Journal: Cancer Treat Rev. 2007 Apr;33(2):161-76. Epub 2007 Jan 22.

Abstract Link: http://www.medifocus.com/abstracts.php?gid=HM009&ID=17240533

128.

Rituximab and its role as maintenance therapy in non-Hodgkin lymphoma.

Authors: Collins-Burow B; Santos ES

Institution: Tulane University School of Medicine, Division of Hematology-Medical Oncology, Tulane Cancer Center, 1430 Tulane Avenue, SL-78, New Orleans, LA 70112, USA. bcollin1@tulane.edu

Journal: Expert Rev Anticancer Ther. 2007 Mar;7(3):257-73.

Abstract Link: http://www.medifocus.com/abstracts.php?gid=HM009&ID=17338647

129.

Pixantrone: a novel aza-anthracenedione in the treatment of non-Hodgkin's lymphomas.

Authors: El-Helw LM; Hancock BW

Institution: Weston Park Hospital, YCR Academic Unit of Clinical Oncology, Sheffield, S10 2SJ, UK.

Journal: Expert Opin Investig Drugs. 2007 Oct;16(10):1683-91.

Abstract Link: http://www.medifocus.com/abstracts.php?gid=HM009&ID=17922631

Go to http://www.medifocus.com/links/HM009/0212 for direct online access to the above Abstract Links.

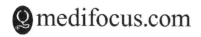

130.

Monoclonal antibodies in the treatment of non-Hodgkin's lymphoma.

Authors:	Fanale MA; Younes A
Institution:	Department of Lymphoma/Myeloma, The University of Texas M.D. Anderson Cancer Center, Houston, Texas, USA. mfanale@mdanderson.org
Journal:	Drugs. 2007;67(3):333-50.
Abstract Link:	http://www.medifocus.com/abstracts.php?gid=HM009&ID=17335294

131.

BiovaxID: a personalized therapeutic cancer vaccine for non-Hodgkin's lymphoma.

Authors:	Lee ST; Jiang YF; Park KU; Woo AF; Neelapu SS
Institution:	The University of Texas M. D. Anderson Cancer Center, Department of Lymphoma and Myeloma, Division of Cancer Medicine, 1515 Holcombe Blvd, Unit 903, Houston, TX, 77030 USA. stlee@mdanderson.org
Journal:	Expert Opin Biol Ther. 2007 Jan;7(1):113-22.
Abstract Link:	http://www.medifocus.com/abstracts.php?gid=HM009&ID=17150023

132.

Drug evaluation: FavId, a patient-specific idiotypic vaccine for non-Hodgkin's lymphoma.

Author:	Reinis M
Institution:	Academy of Sciences of the Czech Republic, Institute of Molecular Genetics, Videnska 1083, Prague 4, CZ-14220, Czech Republic. reinis@img.cas.cz
Journal:	Curr Opin Mol Ther. 2007 Jun;9(3):291-8.
Abstract Link:	http://www.medifocus.com/abstracts.php?gid=HM009&ID=17608028

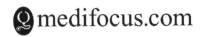 medifocus.com

Clinical Trials Articles

133.

Gem-(R)CHOP versus (R)CHOP: a randomized phase II study of gemcitabine combined with (R)CHOP in untreated aggressive non-Hodgkin's lymphoma--EORTC lymphoma group protocol 20021 (EudraCT number 2004-004635-54).

Authors:	Aurer I; Eghbali H; Raemaekers J; Khaled HM; Fortpied C; Baila L; van der Maazen RW
Institution:	Division of Hematology, Department of Internal Medicine, University Hospital Center Zagreb, Kispaticeva 12, Zagreb, Croatia. aurer@mef.hr
Journal:	Eur J Haematol. 2011 Feb;86(2):111-6. doi: 10.1111/j.1600-0609.2010.01540.x. Epub 2010 Dec 22.
Abstract Link:	http://www.medifocus.com/abstracts.php?gid=HM009&ID=20942843

134.

The differential effect of lenalidomide monotherapy in patients with relapsed or refractory transformed non-Hodgkin lymphoma of distinct histological origin.

Authors:	Czuczman MS; Vose JM; Witzig TE; Zinzani PL; Buckstein R; Polikoff J; Li J; Pietronigro D; Ervin-Haynes A; Reeder CB
Institution:	Roswell Park Cancer Institute, Buffalo, NY 14263, USA. myron.czuczman@roswellpark.org
Journal:	Br J Haematol. 2011 Aug;154(4):477-81. doi: 10.1111/j.1365-2141.2011.08781.x. Epub 2011 Jun 28.
Abstract Link:	http://www.medifocus.com/abstracts.php?gid=HM009&ID=21707581

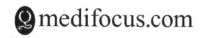

135.

Immunochemotherapy with rituximab, methotrexate, procarbazine, and lomustine for primary CNS lymphoma (PCNSL) in the elderly.

Authors:	Fritsch K; Kasenda B; Hader C; Nikkhah G; Prinz M; Haug V; Haug S; Ihorst G; Finke J; Illerhaus G
Institution:	Department of Hematology and Oncology, Freiburg University Medical Center, Freiburg, Germany.
Journal:	Ann Oncol. 2011 Sep;22(9):2080-5. Epub 2011 Feb 8.
Abstract Link:	http://www.medifocus.com/abstracts.php?gid=HM009&ID=21303800

136.

Autologous peripheral blood stem cell transplantation in children with refractory or relapsed lymphoma: results of Children's Oncology Group study A5962.

Authors:	Harris RE; Termuhlen AM; Smith LM; Lynch J; Henry MM; Perkins SL; Gross TG; Warkentin P; Vlachos A; Harrison L; Cairo MS
Institution:	Division of Bone Marrow Transplant and Immune Deficiency, Cincinnati Children's Hospital Medical Center, Cincinnati, Ohio, USA. Richard.Harris@CCHMC.org
Journal:	Biol Blood Marrow Transplant. 2011 Feb;17(2):249-58. Epub 2010 Jul 15.
Abstract Link:	http://www.medifocus.com/abstracts.php?gid=HM009&ID=20637881

137.

BEAM or BuCyE high-dose chemotherapy followed by autologous stem cell transplantation in non-Hodgkin's lymphoma patients: a single center comparative analysis of efficacy and toxicity.

Authors:	Kim JE; Lee DH; Yoo C; Kim S; Kim SW; Lee JS; Park CJ; Huh J; Suh C
Institution:	Department of Oncology, Asan Medical Center, University of Ulsan College of Medicine, 86 Asan byeongwon-gil, Songpa-gu, 138-736 Seoul, Republic of Korea.
Journal:	Leuk Res. 2011 Feb;35(2):183-7. Epub 2010 Aug 3.
Abstract Link:	http://www.medifocus.com/abstracts.php?gid=HM009&ID=20684990

Go to http://www.medifocus.com/links/HM009/0212 for direct online access to the above Abstract Links.

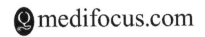

138.

CHOD/BVAM chemotherapy and whole-brain radiotherapy for newly diagnosed primary central nervous system lymphoma.

Authors:	Laack NN; O'Neill BP; Ballman KV; O'Fallon JR; Carrero XW; Kurtin PJ; Scheithauer BW; Brown PD; Habermann TM; Colgan JP; Gilbert MR; Hawkins RB; Morton RF; Windschitl HE; Fitch TR; Pajon ER Jr
Institution:	Department of Radiation Oncology, Mayo Clinic and Mayo Foundation, Rochester, Minnesota 55905, USA.
Journal:	Int J Radiat Oncol Biol Phys. 2011 Oct 1;81(2):476-82. Epub 2010 Aug 26.
Abstract Link:	http://www.medifocus.com/abstracts.php?gid=HM009&ID=20800387

139.

Reduced dose radiotherapy for local control in non-Hodgkin lymphoma: a randomised phase III trial.

Authors:	Lowry L; Smith P; Qian W; Falk S; Benstead K; Illidge T; Linch D; Robinson M; Jack A; Hoskin P
Institution:	Haematology Trials Group, University College London Cancer Trials Centre, UK.
Journal:	Radiother Oncol. 2011 Jul;100(1):86-92. Epub 2011 Jun 12.
Abstract Link:	http://www.medifocus.com/abstracts.php?gid=HM009&ID=21664710

140.

Efficacy and safety of clofarabine in relapsed and/or refractory non-Hodgkin lymphoma, including rituximab-refractory patients.

Authors:	Nabhan C; Davis N; Bitran JD; Galvez A; Fried W; Tolzien K; Foss S; Dewey WM; Venugopal P
Institution:	Division of Hematology and Medical Oncology and Hematology and Oncology Fellowship Program, Advocate Lutheran General Hospital, Park Ridge, IL 60068, USA. Illinois. cnabhan@oncmed.net
Journal:	Cancer. 2011 Apr 1;117(7):1490-7. doi: 10.1002/cncr.25603. Epub 2010 Nov 8.
Abstract Link:	http://www.medifocus.com/abstracts.php?gid=HM009&ID=21425150

Go to http://www.medifocus.com/links/HM009/0212 for direct online access to the above Abstract Links.

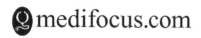

141.

Cladribine combined with rituximab (R-2-CdA) therapy is an effective salvage therapy in relapsed or refractory indolent B-cell non-Hodgkin lymphoma.

Authors:	Nagai H; Ogura M; Kusumoto S; Takahashi N; Yamaguchi M; Takayama N; Kinoshita T; Motoji T; Ohyashiki K; Kosugi H; Matsuda S; Ohnishi K; Omachi K; Hotta T
Institution:	Clinical Research Center, National Hospital Organization Nagoya Medical Center, 4-1-1 Sannomaru, Naka-ku, Nagaoya, Japan. nagaih@nnh.hosp.go.jp
Journal:	Eur J Haematol. 2011 Feb;86(2):117-23. doi: 10.1111/j.1600-0609.2010.01552.x. Epub 2010 Dec 29.
Abstract Link:	http://www.medifocus.com/abstracts.php?gid=HM009&ID=21070370

142.

Phase III trial of CHOP-21 versus CHOP-14 for aggressive non-Hodgkin's lymphoma: final results of the Japan Clinical Oncology Group Study, JCOG 9809.

Authors:	Ohmachi K; Tobinai K; Kobayashi Y; Itoh K; Nakata M; Shibata T; Morishima Y; Ogura M; Suzuki T; Ueda R; Aikawa K; Nakamura S; Fukuda H; Shimoyama M; Hotta T
Institution:	Division of Hematology, Department of Internal Medicine, Tokai University, Isehara, Kanagawa, Japan. 8jmmd004@is.icc.u-tokai.ac.jp
Journal:	Ann Oncol. 2011 Jun;22(6):1382-91. Epub 2010 Dec 31.
Abstract Link:	http://www.medifocus.com/abstracts.php?gid=HM009&ID=21196441

Go to http://www.medifocus.com/links/HM009/0212 for direct online access to the above Abstract Links.

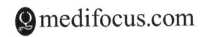
143.

Phase I trial examining addition of gemcitabine to CHOP in intermediate grade NHL.

Authors:	Reagan JL; Rosmarin A; Butera JN; Nadeem A; Schiffman FJ; Sikov WM; Winer E; Mega AE
Institution:	Department of Hematology/Oncology, The Miriam Hospital, 164 Summit Avenue, Providence, RI 02906, USA. jreagan@lifespan.org
Journal:	Cancer Chemother Pharmacol. 2011 Oct;68(4):1075-80. Epub 2011 Jul 15.
Abstract Link:	http://www.medifocus.com/abstracts.php?gid=HM009&ID=21761371

144.

Low-dose radiotherapy in indolent lymphoma.

Authors:	Rossier C; Schick U; Miralbell R; Mirimanoff RO; Weber DC; Ozsahin M
Institution:	Department of Radiation Oncology, Centre Hospitalier Universitaire Vaudois, Lausanne, Switzerland.
Journal:	Int J Radiat Oncol Biol Phys. 2011 Nov 1;81(3):e1-6. Epub 2011 Mar 11.
Abstract Link:	http://www.medifocus.com/abstracts.php?gid=HM009&ID=21398049

145.

A phase I trial of high-dose clofarabine, etoposide, and cyclophosphamide and autologous peripheral blood stem cell transplantation in patients with primary refractory and relapsed and refractory non-Hodgkin lymphoma.

Authors:	Srivastava S; Jones D; Wood LL; Schwartz JE; Nelson RP Jr; Abonour R; Secrest A; Cox E; Baute J; Sullivan C; Kane K; Robertson MJ; Farag SS
Institution:	Department of Medicine, Indiana University School of Medicine, Indianapolis, Indiana 46202, USA.
Journal:	Biol Blood Marrow Transplant. 2011 Jul;17(7):987-94. Epub 2010 Oct 20.
Abstract Link:	http://www.medifocus.com/abstracts.php?gid=HM009&ID=20965266

Go to http://www.medifocus.com/links/HM009/0212 for direct online access to the above Abstract Links.

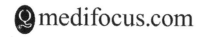

146.

Pixantrone dimaleate in combination with fludarabine, dexamethasone, and rituximab in patients with relapsed or refractory indolent non-Hodgkin lymphoma: phase 1 study with a dose-expansion cohort.

Authors: Srokowski TP; Liebmann JE; Modiano MR; Cohen GI; Pro B; Romaguera JE; Kuepfer C; Singer JW; Fayad LE

Institution: Department of Lymphoma and Myeloma, University of Texas MD Anderson Cancer Center, Houston, Texas, USA.

Journal: Cancer. 2011 Nov 15;117(22):5067-73. doi: 10.1002/cncr.26121. Epub 2011 Jun 16.

Abstract Link: http://www.medifocus.com/abstracts.php?gid=HM009&ID=21681734

147.

A phase II trial of the oral mTOR inhibitor everolimus in relapsed aggressive lymphoma.

Authors: Witzig TE; Reeder CB; LaPlant BR; Gupta M; Johnston PB; Micallef IN; Porrata LF; Ansell SM; Colgan JP; Jacobsen ED; Ghobrial IM; Habermann TM

Institution: Division of Hematology, Department of Medicine, Mayo Clinic College of Medicine and Mayo Foundation, Rochester, MN 55905, USA. Witzig@mayo.edu

Journal: Leukemia. 2011 Feb;25(2):341-7. Epub 2010 Dec 7.

Abstract Link: http://www.medifocus.com/abstracts.php?gid=HM009&ID=21135857

148.

Safety and preliminary efficacy of plerixafor (Mozobil) in combination with chemotherapy and G-CSF: an open-label, multicenter, exploratory trial in patients with multiple myeloma and non-Hodgkin's lymphoma undergoing stem cell mobilization.

Authors: Dugan MJ; Maziarz RT; Bensinger WI; Nademanee A; Liesveld J; Badel K; Dehner C; Gibney C; Bridger G; Calandra G

Institution: Indiana Blood & Marrow Transplantation, Indianapolis, IN 46107, USA. mdugan@ibmtindy.com

Journal: Bone Marrow Transplant. 2010 Jan;45(1):39-47. Epub 2009 Jun 1.

Abstract Link: http://www.medifocus.com/abstracts.php?gid=HM009&ID=19483760

Go to http://www.medifocus.com/links/HM009/0212 for direct online access to the above Abstract Links.

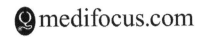

149.

Dose-dense therapy improves survival in aggressive non-Hodgkin's lymphoma.

Authors:	Fridrik MA; Hausmaninger H; Lang A; Drach J; Krieger O; Geissler D; Michlmayr G; Ulsperger E; Chott A; Oberaigner W; Greil R
Institution:	Department Internal Medicine 3, Centre for Hematology and Medical Oncology, General Hospital Linz, Krankenhausstrasse 9, 4020, Linz, Austria. michael.fridrik@akh.linz.at
Journal:	Ann Hematol. 2010 Mar;89(3):273-82. Epub 2009 Aug 20.
Abstract Link:	http://www.medifocus.com/abstracts.php?gid=HM009&ID=19693500

150.

Smoking, alcohol use, obesity, and overall survival from non-Hodgkin lymphoma: a population-based study.

Authors:	Geyer SM; Morton LM; Habermann TM; Allmer C; Davis S; Cozen W; Severson RK; Lynch CF; Wang SS; Maurer MJ; Hartge P; Cerhan JR
Institution:	Department of Health Sciences Research, College of Medicine, Mayo Clinic, Rochester, MN 55905, USA.
Journal:	Cancer. 2010 Jun 15;116(12):2993-3000.
Abstract Link:	http://www.medifocus.com/abstracts.php?gid=HM009&ID=20564404

151.

Phase II study of autologous stem cell transplant using busulfan-melphalan chemotherapy-only conditioning followed by interferon for relapsed poor prognosis follicular non-Hodgkin lymphoma.

Authors:	Grigg AP; Stone J; Milner AD; Schwarer AP; Wolf M; Prince HM; Seymour J; Gill D; Ellis D; Bashford J
Institution:	Department of Clinical Haematology and Bone Marrow Transplantation, Royal Melbourne Hospital and University of Melbourne, Melbourne, Australia. Andrew.grigg@mh.org.au
Journal:	Leuk Lymphoma. 2010 Apr;51(4):641-9.
Abstract Link:	http://www.medifocus.com/abstracts.php?gid=HM009&ID=20218809

Go to http://www.medifocus.com/links/HM009/0212 for direct online access to the above Abstract Links.

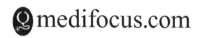

152.

Hematopoietic stem cell transplantation for refractory or recurrent non-Hodgkin lymphoma in children and adolescents.

Authors:	Gross TG; Hale GA; He W; Camitta BM; Sanders JE; Cairo MS; Hayashi RJ; Termuhlen AM; Zhang MJ; Davies SM; Eapen M
Institution:	Department of Pediatrics, Nationwide Children's Hospital, Ohio State University, Columbus, Ohio 43205, USA. thomas.gross@nationwidechildrens.org
Journal:	Biol Blood Marrow Transplant. 2010 Feb;16(2):223-30. Epub 2009 Sep 30.
Abstract Link:	http://www.medifocus.com/abstracts.php?gid=HM009&ID=19800015

153.

Cyclophosphamide, vincristine, and prednisone followed by tositumomab and iodine-131-tositumomab in patients with untreated low-grade follicular lymphoma: eight-year follow-up of a multicenter phase II study.

Authors:	Link BK; Martin P; Kaminski MS; Goldsmith SJ; Coleman M; Leonard JP
Institution:	University of Iowa Hospitals and Clinics, Iowa City, IA, USA.
Journal:	J Clin Oncol. 2010 Jun 20;28(18):3035-41. Epub 2010 May 10.
Abstract Link:	http://www.medifocus.com/abstracts.php?gid=HM009&ID=20458031

154.

Weekly treatment with a combination of bortezomib and bendamustine in relapsed or refractory indolent non-Hodgkin lymphoma.

Authors:	Moosmann P; Heizmann M; Kotrubczik N; Wernli M; Bargetzi M
Journal:	Leuk Lymphoma. 2010 Jan;51(1):149-52.
Abstract Link:	**ABSTRACT NOT AVAILABLE**

Go to http://www.medifocus.com/links/HM009/0212 for direct online access to the above Abstract Links.

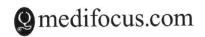

155.

High rates of durable responses with anti-CD22 fractionated radioimmunotherapy: results of a multicenter, phase I/II study in non-Hodgkin's lymphoma.

Authors:	Morschhauser F; Kraeber-Bodere F; Wegener WA; Harousseau JL; Petillon MO; Huglo D; Trumper LH; Meller J; Pfreundschuh M; Kirsch CM; Naumann R; Kropp J; Horne H; Teoh N; Le Gouill S; Bodet-Milin C; Chatal JF; Goldenberg DM
Institution:	Service des Maladies du Sang, Centre Hospitalier Regional, L'Universitaire de Lille, France.
Journal:	J Clin Oncol. 2010 Aug 10;28(23):3709-16. Epub 2010 Jul 12.
Abstract Link:	http://www.medifocus.com/abstracts.php?gid=HM009&ID=20625137

156.

A randomized controlled multicenter study comparing recombinant interleukin 2 (rIL-2) in conjunction with recombinant interferon alpha (IFN-alpha) versus no immunotherapy for patients with malignant lymphoma postautologous stem cell transplantation.

Authors:	Nagler A; Berger R; Ackerstein A; Czyz JA; Diez-Martin JL; Naparstek E; Or R; Gan S; Shimoni A; Slavin S
Institution:	Institute of Hematology, Tel Hashomer, Israel. arnon.nagler@sheba.health.gov.il
Journal:	J Immunother. 2010 Apr;33(3):326-33.
Abstract Link:	http://www.medifocus.com/abstracts.php?gid=HM009&ID=20445353

157.

Phase II study of immunomodulation with granulocyte-macrophage colony-stimulating factor, interleukin-2, and rituximab following autologous stem cell transplant in patients with relapsed or refractory lymphomas.

Authors:	Poire X; Kline J; Grinblatt D; Zimmerman T; Conner K; Muhs C; Gajewski T; Van Besien K; Smith SM
Institution:	Department of Medicine, University of Chicago Medical Center, Chicago, IL 60637, USA.

Go to http://www.medifocus.com/links/HM009/0212 for direct online access to the above Abstract Links.

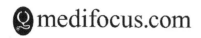

Journal:	Leuk Lymphoma. 2010 Jul;51(7):1241-50.
Abstract Link:	http://www.medifocus.com/abstracts.php?gid=HM009&ID=20496994

158.

Pegfilgrastim appears equivalent to daily dosing of filgrastim to treat neutropenia after autologous peripheral blood stem cell transplantation in patients with non-Hodgkin lymphoma.

Authors:	Rifkin R; Spitzer G; Orloff G; Mandanas R; McGaughey D; Zhan F; Boehm KA; Asmar L; Beveridge R
Institution:	Blood and Marrow Transplant Network, US Oncology Research, Inc, The Woodlands, TX, USA. robert.rifkin@usoncology.com
Journal:	Clin Lymphoma Myeloma Leuk. 2010 Jun;10(3):186-91.
Abstract Link:	http://www.medifocus.com/abstracts.php?gid=HM009&ID=20511163

159.

Primary central nervous system lymphoma in the elderly: a multicentre retrospective analysis.

Authors:	Schuurmans M; Bromberg JE; Doorduijn J; Poortmans P; Taphoorn MJ; Seute T; Enting R; van Imhoff G; van Norden Y; van den Bent MJ
Institution:	Department of Neuro-Oncology, Daniel den Hoed Cancer Centre, Erasmus MC, Rotterdam, the Netherlands.
Journal:	Br J Haematol. 2010 Oct;151(2):179-84. doi: 10.1111/j.1365-2141.2010.08328.x. Epub 2010 Aug 25.
Abstract Link:	http://www.medifocus.com/abstracts.php?gid=HM009&ID=20738305

160.

Ligustrazine as a salvage agent for patients with relapsed or refractory non-Hodgkin's lymphoma.

Authors:	Yang XG; Jiang C
Institution:	Department of Internal Medicine Oncology, Shandong Cancer Hospital, Shandong Academy of Medical Sciences, Jinan, Shandong 250117, China. zlysxgy@yahoo.com.cn
Journal:	Chin Med J (Engl). 2010 Nov;123(22):3206-11.
Abstract Link:	http://www.medifocus.com/abstracts.php?gid=HM009&ID=21163116

Go to http://www.medifocus.com/links/HM009/0212 for direct online access to the above Abstract Links.

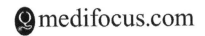
161.

A Phase 1b/2 trial of mapatumumab in patients with relapsed/refractory non-Hodgkin's lymphoma.

Authors: Younes A; Vose JM; Zelenetz AD; Smith MR; Burris HA; Ansell SM; Klein J; Halpern W; Miceli R; Kumm E; Fox NL; Czuczman MS

Institution: MD Anderson Cancer Center, 1515 Holcombe Boulevard, Houston, TX 77030-4009, USA. ayounes@mdanderson.org

Journal: Br J Cancer. 2010 Dec 7;103(12):1783-7. Epub 2010 Nov 16.

Abstract Link: http://www.medifocus.com/abstracts.php?gid=HM009&ID=21081929

162.

Phase I study of the humanized anti-CD40 monoclonal antibody dacetuzumab in refractory or recurrent non-Hodgkin's lymphoma.

Authors: Advani R; Forero-Torres A; Furman RR; Rosenblatt JD; Younes A; Ren H; Harrop K; Whiting N; Drachman JG

Institution: Division of Oncology, Stanford University Medical Center, 875 Blake Wilbur Dr, Stanford, CA 94305, USA. radvani@stanford.edu

Journal: J Clin Oncol. 2009 Sep 10;27(26):4371-7. Epub 2009 Jul 27.

Abstract Link: http://www.medifocus.com/abstracts.php?gid=HM009&ID=19636010

163.

CNS events in elderly patients with aggressive lymphoma treated with modern chemotherapy (CHOP-14) with or without rituximab: an analysis of patients treated in the RICOVER-60 trial of the German High-Grade Non-Hodgkin Lymphoma Study Group (DSHNHL).

Authors: Boehme V; Schmitz N; Zeynalova S; Loeffler M; Pfreundschuh M

Institution: Department of Hematology and Stem Cell Transplantation, Asklepios Hospital St Georg, Hamburg, Germany.

Journal: Blood. 2009 Apr 23;113(17):3896-902. Epub 2009 Jan 14.

Abstract Link: http://www.medifocus.com/abstracts.php?gid=HM009&ID=19144985

Go to http://www.medifocus.com/links/HM009/0212 for direct online access to the above Abstract Links.

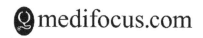

164.

Phase III prospective randomized double-blind placebo-controlled trial of plerixafor plus granulocyte colony-stimulating factor compared with placebo plus granulocyte colony-stimulating factor for autologous stem-cell mobilization and transplantation for patients with non-Hodgkin's lymphoma.

Authors:	DiPersio JF; Micallef IN; Stiff PJ; Bolwell BJ; Maziarz RT; Jacobsen E; Nademanee A; McCarty J; Bridger G; Calandra G
Institution:	Washington University School of Medicine, St Louis, MO, USA. jdipersi@im.wustl.edu
Journal:	J Clin Oncol. 2009 Oct 1;27(28):4767-73. Epub 2009 Aug 31.
Abstract Link:	http://www.medifocus.com/abstracts.php?gid=HM009&ID=19720922

165.

Positron emission tomography guided therapy of aggressive non-Hodgkin lymphomas--the PETAL trial.

Authors:	Duhrsen U; Huttmann A; Jockel KH; Muller S
Institution:	Department of Hematology, University Hospital Essen, University of Duisburg-Essen, Essen, Germany. ulrich.duehrsen@uk-essen.de
Journal:	Leuk Lymphoma. 2009 Nov;50(11):1757-60.
Abstract Link:	http://www.medifocus.com/abstracts.php?gid=HM009&ID=19863177

166.

High-dose cytarabine plus high-dose methotrexate versus high-dose methotrexate alone in patients with primary CNS lymphoma: a randomised phase 2 trial.

Authors:	Ferreri AJ; Reni M; Foppoli M; Martelli M; Pangalis GA; Frezzato M; Cabras MG; Fabbri A; Corazzelli G; Ilariucci F; Rossi G; Soffietti R; Stelitano C; Vallisa D; Zaja F; Zoppegno L; Aondio GM; Avvisati G; Balzarotti M; Brandes AA; Fajardo J; Gomez H; Guarini A; Pinotti G; Rigacci L; Uhlmann C; Picozzi P; Vezzulli P; Ponzoni M; Zucca E; Caligaris-Cappio F; Cavalli F
Institution:	Unit of Lymphoid Malignancies, San Raffaele Scientific Institute, Milan, Italy. andres.ferreri@hsr.it

Go to http://www.medifocus.com/links/HM009/0212 for direct online access to the above Abstract Links.

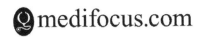
Journal:	Lancet. 2009 Oct 31;374(9700):1512-20. Epub 2009 Sep 18.
Abstract Link:	http://www.medifocus.com/abstracts.php?gid=HM009&ID=19767089

167.

Should intra-cerebrospinal fluid prophylaxis be part of initial therapy for patients with non-Hodgkin lymphoma: what we know, and how we can find out more.

Authors:	Herrlinger U; Glantz M; Schlegel U; Gisselbrecht C; Cavalli F
Institution:	Division of Clinical Neuro-oncology, Department of Neurology, University of Bonn, Bonn, Germany. Ulrich.Herrlinger@ukb.uni-bonn.de
Journal:	Semin Oncol. 2009 Aug;36(4 Suppl 2):S25-34.
Abstract Link:	http://www.medifocus.com/abstracts.php?gid=HM009&ID=19660681

168.

Humanized anti-CD20 antibody, veltuzumab, in refractory/recurrent non-Hodgkin's lymphoma: phase I/II results.

Authors:	Morschhauser F; Leonard JP; Fayad L; Coiffier B; Petillon MO; Coleman M; Schuster SJ; Dyer MJ; Horne H; Teoh N; Wegener WA; Goldenberg DM
Institution:	Service des Maladies du Sang Centre Hospitalier Regional, Lille, France. f-morschhauser@chru-lille.fr
Journal:	J Clin Oncol. 2009 Jul 10;27(20):3346-53. Epub 2009 May 18.
Abstract Link:	http://www.medifocus.com/abstracts.php?gid=HM009&ID=19451441

169.

High-dose therapy and autologous peripheral blood stem cell transplantation as salvage treatment for AIDS-related lymphoma: long-term results of the Italian Cooperative Group on AIDS and Tumors (GICAT) study with analysis of prognostic factors.

Authors:	Re A; Michieli M; Casari S; Allione B; Cattaneo C; Rupolo M; Spina M; Manuele R; Vaccher E; Mazzucato M; Abbruzzese L; Ferremi P; Carosi G; Tirelli U; Rossi G
Institution:	Division of Hematology, Spedali Civili di Brescia, Brescia, Italy. sandrore@aruba.it

Go to http://www.medifocus.com/links/HM009/0212 for direct online access to the above Abstract Links.

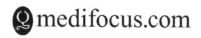

Journal: Blood. 2009 Aug 13;114(7):1306-13. Epub 2009 May 18.
Abstract Link: http://www.medifocus.com/abstracts.php?gid=HM009&ID=19451551

170.

Vincristine sulfate liposomes injection (Marqibo) in heavily pretreated patients with refractory aggressive non-Hodgkin lymphoma: report of the pivotal phase 2 study.

Authors: Rodriguez MA; Pytlik R; Kozak T; Chhanabhai M; Gascoyne R; Lu B; Deitcher SR; Winter JN

Institution: Lymphoma/Myeloma Department, The University of Texas M. D. Anderson Cancer Center, Houston, Texas 77030, USA. marodriguez@mdanderson.org
Journal: Cancer. 2009 Aug 1;115(15):3475-82.
Abstract Link: http://www.medifocus.com/abstracts.php?gid=HM009&ID=19536896

171.

A multicenter phase II trial of etoposide, methylprednisolone, high-dose cytarabine, and oxaliplatin for patients with primary refractory/relapsed aggressive non-Hodgkin's lymphoma.

Authors: Sym SJ; Lee DH; Kang HJ; Nam SH; Kim HY; Kim SJ; Eom HS; Kim WS; Suh C

Institution: Department of Internal Medicine, Asan Medical Center, University of Ulsan College of Medicine, Songpa-gu, Seoul, South Korea.
Journal: Cancer Chemother Pharmacol. 2009 Jun;64(1):27-33. Epub 2008 Oct 7.
Abstract Link: http://www.medifocus.com/abstracts.php?gid=HM009&ID=18839172

Go to http://www.medifocus.com/links/HM009/0212 for direct online access to the above Abstract Links.

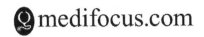

172.

Lenalidomide oral monotherapy produces durable responses in relapsed or refractory indolent non-Hodgkin's Lymphoma.

Authors: Witzig TE; Wiernik PH; Moore T; Reeder C; Cole C; Justice G; Kaplan H; Voralia M; Pietronigro D; Takeshita K; Ervin-Haynes A; Zeldis JB; Vose JM

Institution: Mayo Clinic, Rochester, MN 55905, USA. witzig@mayo.edu
Journal: J Clin Oncol. 2009 Nov 10;27(32):5404-9. Epub 2009 Oct 5.
Abstract Link: http://www.medifocus.com/abstracts.php?gid=HM009&ID=19805688

173.

Bendamustine in patients with rituximab-refractory indolent and transformed non-Hodgkin's lymphoma: results from a phase II multicenter, single-agent study.

Authors: Friedberg JW; Cohen P; Chen L; Robinson KS; Forero-Torres A; La Casce AS; Fayad LE; Bessudo A; Camacho ES; Williams ME; van der Jagt RH; Oliver JW; Cheson BD

Institution: James P. Wilmot Cancer Center, University of Rochester, 601 Elmwood Ave, Box 704, Rochester, NY, 14642, USA. Jonathan_Friedberg@URMC.Rochester.edu
Journal: J Clin Oncol. 2008 Jan 10;26(2):204-10.
Abstract Link: http://www.medifocus.com/abstracts.php?gid=HM009&ID=18182663

174.

A revisit of prophylactic lamivudine for chemotherapy-associated hepatitis B reactivation in non-Hodgkin's lymphoma: a randomized trial.

Authors: Hsu C; Hsiung CA; Su IJ; Hwang WS; Wang MC; Lin SF; Lin TH; Hsiao HH; Young JH; Chang MC; Liao YM; Li CC; Wu HB; Tien HF; Chao TY; Liu TW; Cheng AL; Chen PJ

Institution: Department of Oncology, National Taiwan University Hospital, Taipei, Taiwan.
Journal: Hepatology. 2008 Mar;47(3):844-53.
Abstract Link: http://www.medifocus.com/abstracts.php?gid=HM009&ID=18302293

Go to http://www.medifocus.com/links/HM009/0212 for direct online access to the above Abstract Links.

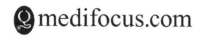

175.

Primary central nervous system lymphoma: monocenter, long-term, intent-to-treat analysis.

Authors: Kiewe P; Fischer L; Martus P; Thiel E; Korfel A

Institution: Department of Hematology, Oncology, and Transfusion Medicine, Charite Universitatsmedizin Berlin, Campus Benjamin Franklin, Berlin, Germany. philipp.kiewe@charite.de

Journal: Cancer. 2008 Apr 15;112(8):1812-20.

Abstract Link: http://www.medifocus.com/abstracts.php?gid=HM009&ID=18318432

176.

Phase II trial of a transplantation regimen of yttrium-90 ibritumomab tiuxetan and high-dose chemotherapy in patients with non-Hodgkin's lymphoma.

Authors: Krishnan A; Nademanee A; Fung HC; Raubitschek AA; Molina A; Yamauchi D; Rodriguez R; Spielberger RT; Falk P; Palmer JM; Forman SJ

Institution: Division of Hematology and Hematopoietic Cell Transplantation, City of Hope Comprehensive Cancer Center, Duarte, CA 91010, USA. akrishnan@coh.org

Journal: J Clin Oncol. 2008 Jan 1;26(1):90-5. Epub 2007 Nov 19.

Abstract Link: http://www.medifocus.com/abstracts.php?gid=HM009&ID=18025438

177.

A multicentre phase II clinical experience with the novel aza-epothilone Ixabepilone (BMS247550) in patients with relapsed or refractory indolent non-Hodgkin lymphoma and mantle cell lymphoma.

Authors: O'Connor OA; Portlock C; Moskowitz C; Straus D; Hamlin P; Stubblefield M; Dumetrescu O; Colevas AD; Grant B; Zelenetz A

Institution: Department of Medicine, Division of Hematologic Oncology, Memorial Sloan Kettering Cancer Center, Lymphoma Service, New York, NY 10032, USA. oo2130@columbia.edu

Journal: Br J Haematol. 2008 Oct;143(2):201-9. Epub 2008 Aug 4.

Abstract Link: http://www.medifocus.com/abstracts.php?gid=HM009&ID=18691173

Go to http://www.medifocus.com/links/HM009/0212 for direct online access to the above Abstract Links.

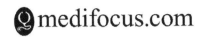

178.

Dose-escalated CHOEP for the treatment of young patients with aggressive non-Hodgkin's lymphoma: II. Results of the randomized high-CHOEP trial of the German High-Grade Non-Hodgkin's Lymphoma Study Group (DSHNHL).

Authors:	Pfreundschuh M; Zwick C; Zeynalova S; Duhrsen U; Pfluger KH; Vrieling T; Mesters R; Mergenthaler HG; Einsele H; Bentz M; Lengfelder E; Trumper L; Rube C; Schmitz N; Loeffler M
Institution:	Saarland University Medical School, Homburg, Germany. inmpfr@uniklinikum-saarland.de
Journal:	Ann Oncol. 2008 Mar;19(3):545-52. Epub 2007 Dec 6.
Abstract Link:	http://www.medifocus.com/abstracts.php?gid=HM009&ID=18065407

179.

Nonmyeloablative allogeneic hematopoietic cell transplantation in relapsed, refractory, and transformed indolent non-Hodgkin's lymphoma.

Authors:	Rezvani AR; Storer B; Maris M; Sorror ML; Agura E; Maziarz RT; Wade JC; Chauncey T; Forman SJ; Lange T; Shizuru J; Langston A; Pulsipher MA; Sandmaier BM; Storb R; Maloney DG
Institution:	Fred Hutchinson Cancer Research Center, 1100 Fairview Ave N, MS D1-100, Seattle, WA 98109, USA.
Journal:	J Clin Oncol. 2008 Jan 10;26(2):211-7. Epub 2007 Dec 3.
Abstract Link:	http://www.medifocus.com/abstracts.php?gid=HM009&ID=18056679

180.

A phase 2 pilot study of pegfilgrastim and filgrastim for mobilizing peripheral blood progenitor cells in patients with non-Hodgkin's lymphoma receiving chemotherapy.

Authors:	Russell N; Mesters R; Schubert J; Boogaerts M; Johnsen HE; Canizo CD; Baker N; Barker P; Skacel T; Schmitz N
Institution:	Department of Hematology, Nottingham University Hospitals NHS Trust (City Campus), Nottingham NG5 1PB, United Kingdom. nigel.russell@nottingham.ac.uk

Go to http://www.medifocus.com/links/HM009/0212 for direct online access to the above Abstract Links.

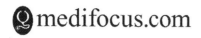medifocus.com

| Journal: | Haematologica. 2008 Mar;93(3):405-12. Epub 2008 Feb 11. |
| Abstract Link: | http://www.medifocus.com/abstracts.php?gid=HM009&ID=18268285 |

181.

Total body irradiation, etoposide, cyclophosphamide, and autologous peripheral blood stem-cell transplantation followed by randomization to therapy with interleukin-2 versus observation for patients with non-Hodgkin lymphoma: results of a phase 3 randomized trial by the Southwest Oncology Group (SWOG 9438).

Authors:	Thompson JA; Fisher RI; Leblanc M; Forman SJ; Press OW; Unger JM; Nademanee AP; Stiff PJ; Petersdorf SH; Fefer A
Institution:	Puget Sound Oncology Consortium, Seattle, WA, USA. jat@u.washington.edu
Journal:	Blood. 2008 Apr 15;111(8):4048-54. Epub 2008 Feb 6.
Abstract Link:	http://www.medifocus.com/abstracts.php?gid=HM009&ID=18256325

182.

Dose-escalated CHOEP for the treatment of young patients with aggressive non-Hodgkin's lymphoma: I. A randomized dose escalation and feasibility study with bi- and tri-weekly regimens.

Authors:	Trumper L; Zwick C; Ziepert M; Hohloch K; Schmits R; Mohren M; Liersch R; Bentz M; Graeven U; Wruck U; Hoffmann M; Metzner B; Hasenclever D; Loeffler M; Pfreundschuh M
Institution:	Hematology and Oncology, University Hospital Gottingen, Germany.
Journal:	Ann Oncol. 2008 Mar;19(3):538-44. Epub 2008 Jan 22.
Abstract Link:	http://www.medifocus.com/abstracts.php?gid=HM009&ID=18212092

Go to http://www.medifocus.com/links/HM009/0212 for direct online access to the above Abstract Links.

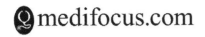

183.

Lenalidomide monotherapy in relapsed or refractory aggressive non-Hodgkin's lymphoma.

Authors:	Wiernik PH; Lossos IS; Tuscano JM; Justice G; Vose JM; Cole CE; Lam W; McBride K; Wride K; Pietronigro D; Takeshita K; Ervin-Haynes A; Zeldis JB; Habermann TM
Institution:	Our Lady of Mercy Cancer Center, New York Medical College, Bronx, NY, USA.
Journal:	J Clin Oncol. 2008 Oct 20;26(30):4952-7. Epub 2008 Jul 7.
Abstract Link:	http://www.medifocus.com/abstracts.php?gid=HM009&ID=18606983

184.

Equitoxicity of bolus and infusional etoposide: results of a multicenter randomised trial of the German High-Grade Non-Hodgkins Lymphoma Study Group (DSHNHL) in elderly patients with refractory or relapsing aggressive non-Hodgkin lymphoma using the CEMP regimen (cisplatinum, etoposide, mitoxantrone and prednisone).

Authors:	Zwick C; Birkmann J; Peter N; Bodenstein H; Fuchs R; Hanel M; Reiser M; Hensel M; Clemens M; Zeynalova S; Ziepert M; Pfreundschuh M
Institution:	Innere Medizin I, Universitatskliniken des Saarlandes, Homburg, Germany.
Journal:	Ann Hematol. 2008 Sep;87(9):717-26. Epub 2008 Jun 28.
Abstract Link:	http://www.medifocus.com/abstracts.php?gid=HM009&ID=18587579

185.

Variations in chemotherapy and radiation therapy in a large nationwide and community-based cohort of elderly patients with non-Hodgkin lymphoma.

Authors:	Berrios-Rivera JP; Fang S; Cabanillas ME; Cabanillas F; Lu H; Du XL
Institution:	Division of Epidemiology, University of Texas School of Public Health, Houston, Texas 77030, USA.
Journal:	Am J Clin Oncol. 2007 Apr;30(2):163-71.
Abstract Link:	http://www.medifocus.com/abstracts.php?gid=HM009&ID=17414466

Go to http://www.medifocus.com/links/HM009/0212 for direct online access to the above Abstract Links.

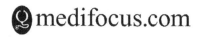

186.

Ifosphamide, etoposide and epirubicin is an effective combined salvage and peripheral blood stem cell mobilisation regimen for transplant-eligible patients with non-Hodgkin lymphoma and Hodgkin disease.

Authors: Bishton MJ; Lush RJ; Byrne JL; Russell NH; Shaw BE; Haynes AP
Institution: Department of Haematology, Nottingham City Hospital, Nottingham, UK. mj_bishton@hotmail.com
Journal: Br J Haematol. 2007 Mar;136(5):752-61.
Abstract Link: http://www.medifocus.com/abstracts.php?gid=HM009&ID=17313378

187.

A phase I/IIa clinical trial of CLAOP21 and CLAOP14 in patients with high grade non-Hodgkins lymphoma.

Authors: Busse A; Hutter G; Siehl JM; Schmittel A; Thiel E; Keilholz U
Institution: Department of Medicine III, Charite, Campus Benjamin Franklin, Berlin, Germany.
Journal: Leuk Lymphoma. 2007 Sep;48(9):1755-63.
Abstract Link: http://www.medifocus.com/abstracts.php?gid=HM009&ID=17786711

188.

Phase II trial of the combination of denileukin diftitox and rituximab for relapsed/refractory B-cell non-Hodgkin lymphoma.

Authors: Dang NH; Fayad L; McLaughlin P; Romaguara JE; Hagemeister F; Goy A; Neelapu S; Samaniego F; Walker PL; Wang M; Rodriguez MA; Tong AT; Pro B
Institution: Department of Hematologic Malignancies, Nevada Cancer Institute, Las Vegas, NV 89135, USA. ndang@nvcancer.org
Journal: Br J Haematol. 2007 Aug;138(4):502-5. Epub 2007 Jun 29.
Abstract Link: http://www.medifocus.com/abstracts.php?gid=HM009&ID=17608763

Go to http://www.medifocus.com/links/HM009/0212 for direct online access to the above Abstract Links.

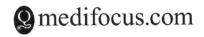

189.

Low-dose oral fludarabine plus cyclophosphamide as first-line treatment in elderly patients with indolent non-Hodgkin lymphoma.

Authors:	Fabbri A; Lenoci M; Gozzetti A; Chitarrelli I; Olcese F; Raspadori D; Gobbi M; Lauria F
Institution:	Unit of Haematology and Transplants, Policlinico S Maria alle Scotte, University of Siena, Siena, Italy. fabbri7@unisi.it
Journal:	Br J Haematol. 2007 Oct;139(1):90-3.
Abstract Link:	http://www.medifocus.com/abstracts.php?gid=HM009&ID=17854311

190.

AMD3100 affects autograft lymphocyte collection and progression-free survival after autologous stem cell transplantation in non-Hodgkin lymphoma.

Authors:	Holtan SG; Porrata LF; Micallef IN; Padley DJ; Inwards DJ; Ansell SA; Johnston PB; Gastineau DA; Markovic SN
Institution:	Department of Medicine, Mayo Clinic College of Medicine, Rochester, MN 55905, USA.
Journal:	Clin Lymphoma Myeloma. 2007 Jan;7(4):315-8.
Abstract Link:	http://www.medifocus.com/abstracts.php?gid=HM009&ID=17324341

191.

Phase II study of denileukin diftitox for previously treated indolent non-Hodgkin lymphoma: final results of E1497.

Authors:	Kuzel TM; Li S; Eklund J; Foss F; Gascoyne R; Abramson N; Schwerkoske JF; Weller E; Horning SJ
Institution:	Feinberg School of Medicine-Northwestern University, Chicago, IL 60611, USA. t-kuzel@northwestern.edu
Journal:	Leuk Lymphoma. 2007 Dec;48(12):2397-402. Epub 2007 Oct 13.
Abstract Link:	http://www.medifocus.com/abstracts.php?gid=HM009&ID=17943599

Go to http://www.medifocus.com/links/HM009/0212 for direct online access to the above Abstract Links.

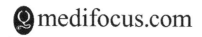

192.

Dose-attenuated radioimmunotherapy with tositumomab and iodine 131 tositumomab in patients with recurrent non-Hodgkin's lymphoma (NHL) and extensive bone marrow involvement.

Authors:	Mones JV; Coleman M; Kostakoglu L; Furman RR; Chadburn A; Shore TB; Muss D; Stewart P; Kroll S; Vallabhajosula S; Goldsmith SJ; Leonard JP
Institution:	Center for Lymphoma and Myeloma, Division of Hematology/Oncology, Weill Medical College of Cornell University and New York Presbyterian Hospital, New York, NY 10021, USA.
Journal:	Leuk Lymphoma. 2007 Feb;48(2):342-8.
Abstract Link:	http://www.medifocus.com/abstracts.php?gid=HM009&ID=17325895

193.

Allogeneic stem cell transplantation with T cell-depleted grafts for lymphoproliferative malignancies.

Authors:	Novitzky N; Thomas V
Institution:	University of Cape Town Leukaemia Centre and Department of Haematology, Groote Schuur Hospital, Cape Town, Western Cape, South Africa. novitzky@cormack.uct.ac.za
Journal:	Biol Blood Marrow Transplant. 2007 Jan;13(1):107-15.
Abstract Link:	http://www.medifocus.com/abstracts.php?gid=HM009&ID=17222759

194.

Effect of cytomegalovirus prophylaxis with immunoglobulin or with antiviral drugs on post-transplant non-Hodgkin lymphoma: a multicentre retrospective analysis.

Authors:	Opelz G; Daniel V; Naujokat C; Fickenscher H; Dohler B
Institution:	Department of Transplantation Immunology, Institute of Immunology, University of Heidelberg, Heidelberg, Germany. gerhard.opelz@med.uni-heidelberg.de
Journal:	Lancet Oncol. 2007 Mar;8(3):212-8.
Abstract Link:	http://www.medifocus.com/abstracts.php?gid=HM009&ID=17329191

Go to http://www.medifocus.com/links/HM009/0212 for direct online access to the above Abstract Links.

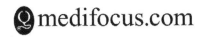

195.

Phase II study of three dose levels of continuous erythropoietin receptor activator (C.E.R.A.) in anaemic patients with aggressive non-Hodgkin's lymphoma receiving combination chemotherapy.

Authors:	Osterborg A; Steegmann JL; Hellmann A; Couban S; Mayer J; Eid JE
Institution:	Departments of Oncology and Haematology, Karolinska University Hospital, Stockholm, Sweden. anders.osterborg@karolinska.se
Journal:	Br J Haematol. 2007 Mar;136(5):736-44.
Abstract Link:	http://www.medifocus.com/abstracts.php?gid=HM009&ID=17313376

196.

High dose CHOP: A phase II study of initial treatment in aggressive non-Hodgkin lymphoma. Cancer and Leukemia Group B 9351.

Authors:	Peterson BA; Johnson J; Shipp MA; Barcos M; Gockerman JP; Canellos GP; Cancer FT; Leukemia GB
Institution:	University of Minnesota. Minneapolis, MN. USA.
Journal:	Leuk Lymphoma. 2007 May;48(5):870-80.
Abstract Link:	http://www.medifocus.com/abstracts.php?gid=HM009&ID=17487729

197.

Phase I study of intraventricular administration of rituximab in patients with recurrent CNS and intraocular lymphoma.

Authors:	Rubenstein JL; Fridlyand J; Abrey L; Shen A; Karch J; Wang E; Issa S; Damon L; Prados M; McDermott M; O'Brien J; Haqq C; Shuman M
Institution:	Division of Hematology/Oncology, and the Department of Epidemiology and Biostatistics, University of California, San Francisco, San Francisco, CA 94143, USA. jamesr@medicine.ucsf.edu
Journal:	J Clin Oncol. 2007 Apr 10;25(11):1350-6. Epub 2007 Feb 20.
Abstract Link:	http://www.medifocus.com/abstracts.php?gid=HM009&ID=17312328

Go to http://www.medifocus.com/links/HM009/0212 for direct online access to the above Abstract Links.

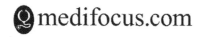
198.

Ifosfamide, etoposide, cytarabine, and dexamethasone as salvage treatment followed by high-dose cyclophosphamide, melphalan, and etoposide with autologous peripheral blood stem cell transplantation for relapsed or refractory lymphomas.

Authors:	Schutt P; Passon J; Ebeling P; Welt A; Muller S; Metz K; Moritz T; Seeber S; Nowrousian MR
Institution:	Department of Internal Medicine (Cancer Research), West German Cancer Center, University of Duisburg-Essen Medical School, Essen, Germany.
Journal:	Eur J Haematol. 2007 Feb;78(2):93-101.
Abstract Link:	http://www.medifocus.com/abstracts.php?gid=HM009&ID=17313557

199.

Yttrium-90-ibritumomab tiuxetan (Zevalin) combined with high-dose BEAM chemotherapy and autologous stem cell transplantation for chemo-refractory aggressive non-Hodgkin's lymphoma.

Authors:	Shimoni A; Zwas ST; Oksman Y; Hardan I; Shem-Tov N; Yerushalmi R; Avigdor A; Ben-Bassat I; Nagler A
Institution:	Division of Hematology and Bone Marrow Transplantation, Chaim Sheba Medical Center, Tel-Hashomer, Israel. ashimoni@sheba.health.gov.il
Journal:	Exp Hematol. 2007 Apr;35(4):534-40.
Abstract Link:	http://www.medifocus.com/abstracts.php?gid=HM009&ID=17379063

200.

Phase II trial of CHOP plus rituximab in patients with HIV-associated non-Hodgkin's lymphoma.

Authors:	Spina M; Simonelli C; Tirelli U
Journal:	J Clin Oncol. 2007 Feb 20;25(6):e7.
Abstract Link:	**ABSTRACT NOT AVAILABLE**

Go to http://www.medifocus.com/links/HM009/0212 for direct online access to the above Abstract Links.

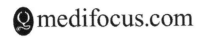

201.

T-cell non-Hodgkin's lymphoma: treatment outcomes and survival in 3 large UK centres.

Authors:	Wright J; Johnson P; Smith P; Horsman JM; Hancock BW
Institution:	Royal Hallamshire Hospital, Sheffield, UK.
Journal:	Acta Haematol. 2007;118(2):123-5. Epub 2007 Sep 4.
Abstract Link:	**ABSTRACT NOT AVAILABLE**

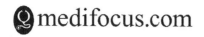

Radiation Therapy Articles

202.

Dexa-BEAM as salvage therapy in patients with primary refractory aggressive non-Hodgkin lymphoma.

Authors:	Atta J; Chow KU; Weidmann E; Mitrou PS; Hoelzer D; Martin H
Institution:	Department of Hematology, J. W. Goethe-University Hospital, Frankfurt, Germany. atta@em.uni-frankfurt.de
Journal:	Leuk Lymphoma. 2007 Feb;48(2):349-56.
Abstract Link:	http://www.medifocus.com/abstracts.php?gid=HM009&ID=17325896

203.

Retreatment with yttrium-90 ibritumomab tiuxetan in patients with B-cell non-Hodgkin's lymphoma.

Authors:	Shah J; Wang W; Harrough VD; Saville W; Meredith R; Shen S; Mueh J; Lister J; Jasthy S; Maggass G; McKay C; Krumdieck R; Tharp M; Winter C; Gregory S; Buchholz W; Awasthi S; Jacobs S; Chung H; Egner J; Lobuglio AF; Forero A
Institution:	Department of Medicine, Division of Hematology/Oncology, University of Alabama at Birmingham Comprehensive Cancer Center, Birmingham, AL, USA.
Journal:	Leuk Lymphoma. 2007 Sep;48(9):1736-44.
Abstract Link:	http://www.medifocus.com/abstracts.php?gid=HM009&ID=17786709

204.

Therapeutic radiation for lymphoma: risk of malignant mesothelioma.

Authors:	Teta MJ; Lau E; Sceurman BK; Wagner ME
Institution:	Exponent, Inc., Health Sciences Practice, New York, New York, USA. jteta@exponent.com
Journal:	Cancer. 2007 Apr 1;109(7):1432-8.
Abstract Link:	http://www.medifocus.com/abstracts.php?gid=HM009&ID=17315168

Go to http://www.medifocus.com/links/HM009/0212 for direct online access to the above Abstract Links.

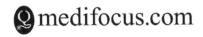
medifocus.com

Stem Cell Transplantation Articles

205.

Allogeneic stem cell transplantation in patients with non-Hodgkin lymphoma who experienced relapse or progression after autologous stem cell transplantation.

Authors:	Kim JW; Kim BS; Bang SM; Kim I; Kim DH; Kim WS; Yang DH; Lee JJ; Lee JH; Kim JS; Sohn SK; Yhim HY; Kwak JY; Yoon SS; Lee JS; Park S; Kim BK
Institution:	Department of Internal Medicine, Seoul National University College of Medicine, 101 Daehak-ro, Jongro-gu, Seoul, 110-744, South Korea.
Journal:	Ann Hematol. 2011 Dec;90(12):1409-18. Epub 2011 Apr 6.
Abstract Link:	http://www.medifocus.com/abstracts.php?gid=HM009&ID=21468694

206.

Allogeneic hematopoietic cell transplant for peripheral T-cell non-Hodgkin lymphoma results in long-term disease control.

Authors:	Zain J; Palmer JM; Delioukina M; Thomas S; Tsai NC; Nademanee A; Popplewell L; Gaal K; Senitzer D; Kogut N; O'Donnell M; Forman SJ
Institution:	Department of Medical Oncology, NYU Medical Center, New York, USA.
Journal:	Leuk Lymphoma. 2011 Aug;52(8):1463-73. Epub 2011 Jun 24.
Abstract Link:	http://www.medifocus.com/abstracts.php?gid=HM009&ID=21699453

207.

Superior survival after replacing oral with intravenous busulfan in autologous stem cell transplantation for non-Hodgkin lymphoma with busulfan, cyclophosphamide and etoposide.

Authors:	Dean RM; Pohlman B; Sweetenham JW; Sobecks RM; Kalaycio ME; Smith SD; Copelan EA; Andresen S; Rybicki LA; Curtis J; Bolwell BJ
Institution:	Taussig Cancer Institute, Cleveland Clinic, OH 44195, USA. deanr@ccf.org
Journal:	Br J Haematol. 2010 Jan;148(2):226-34. Epub 2009 Oct 11.
Abstract Link:	http://www.medifocus.com/abstracts.php?gid=HM009&ID=19821828

Go to http://www.medifocus.com/links/HM009/0212 for direct online access to the above Abstract Links.

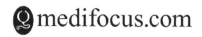

208.

Allogeneic stem cell transplantation for patients with relapsed chemorefractory aggressive non-hodgkin lymphomas.

Authors: Hamadani M; Benson DM Jr; Hofmeister CC; Elder P; Blum W; Porcu P; Garzon R; Blum KA; Lin TS; Marcucci G; Devine SM

Institution: Hematology and Oncology, Arthur G James Comprehensive Cancer Center, The Ohio State University, Columbus, Ohio 43210, USA. mehdi.hamadani@gmail.com

Journal: Biol Blood Marrow Transplant. 2009 May;15(5):547-53. Epub 2009 Mar 9.

Abstract Link: http://www.medifocus.com/abstracts.php?gid=HM009&ID=19361746

209.

Busulfan and cyclophosphamide (Bu/Cy) as a preparative regimen for autologous stem cell transplantation in patients with non-Hodgkin lymphoma: a single-institution experience.

Authors: Ulrickson M; Aldridge J; Kim HT; Hochberg EP; Hammerman P; Dube C; Attar E; Ballen KK; Dey BR; McAfee SL; Spitzer TR; Chen YB

Institution: Department of Hematology/Oncology, Massachusetts General Hospital, Boston, Massachusetts 02114, USA.

Journal: Biol Blood Marrow Transplant. 2009 Nov;15(11):1447-54. Epub 2009 Sep 1.

Abstract Link: http://www.medifocus.com/abstracts.php?gid=HM009&ID=19822305

210.

Unrelated donor hematopoietic cell transplantation for non-hodgkin lymphoma: long-term outcomes.

Authors: van Besien K; Carreras J; Bierman PJ; Logan BR; Molina A; King R; Nelson G; Fay JW; Champlin RE; Lazarus HM; Vose JM; Hari PN

Institution: University of Chicago Medical Center, Chicago, Illinois, USA. kvbesien@uchicago.edu

Journal: Biol Blood Marrow Transplant. 2009 May;15(5):554-63. Epub 2009 Mar 9.

Abstract Link: http://www.medifocus.com/abstracts.php?gid=HM009&ID=19361747

Go to http://www.medifocus.com/links/HM009/0212 for direct online access to the above Abstract Links.

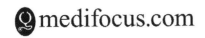

211.

Higher infused CD34+ hematopoietic stem cell dose correlates with earlier lymphocyte recovery and better clinical outcome after autologous stem cell transplantation in non-Hodgkin's lymphoma.

Authors: Yoon DH; Sohn BS; Jang G; Kim EK; Kang BW; Kim C; Kim JE; Kim S; Lee DH; Lee JS; Park SJ; Park CJ; Huh J; Suh C

Institution: Department of Oncology, Laboratory Medicine, and Pathology, Asan Medical Center, University of Ulsan College of Medicine, Seoul, Korea.

Journal: Transfusion. 2009 Sep;49(9):1890-900. Epub 2009 May 11.

Abstract Link: http://www.medifocus.com/abstracts.php?gid=HM009&ID=19453991

212.

Autologous SCT with a dose-reduced BU and CY regimen in older patients with non-Hodgkin's lymphoma.

Authors: Yusuf RZ; Dey B; Yeap BY; McAfee S; Attar E; Sepe PS; Dube C; Spitzer TR; Ballen KK

Institution: Division of Hematology/Oncology, Department of Medicine, Massachusetts General Hospital, Boston, MA 02114, USA.

Journal: Bone Marrow Transplant. 2009 Jan;43(1):37-42. Epub 2008 Sep 15.

Abstract Link: http://www.medifocus.com/abstracts.php?gid=HM009&ID=18794868

213.

Hematopoietic cell transplantation for non-Hodgkin's lymphoma: yesterday, today, and tomorrow.

Author: Appelbaum FR

Journal: J Clin Oncol. 2008 Jun 20;26(18):2927-9.

Abstract Link: **ABSTRACT NOT AVAILABLE**

Go to http://www.medifocus.com/links/HM009/0212 for direct online access to the above Abstract Links.

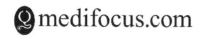

214.

High response rate to donor lymphocyte infusion after allogeneic stem cell transplantation for indolent non-Hodgkin lymphoma.

Authors:	Bloor AJ; Thomson K; Chowdhry N; Verfuerth S; Ings SJ; Chakraverty R; Linch DC; Goldstone AH; Peggs KS; Mackinnon S
Institution:	Department of Haematology, Royal Free and University College London School of Medicine, London, United Kingdom. drbloor@tiscali.co.uk
Journal:	Biol Blood Marrow Transplant. 2008 Jan;14(1):50-8.
Abstract Link:	http://www.medifocus.com/abstracts.php?gid=HM009&ID=18158961

215.

Time-dependent effect of non-Hodgkin's lymphoma grade on disease-free survival of relapsed/refractory patients treated with high-dose chemotherapy plus autotransplantation.

Authors:	Fu P; van Heeckeren WJ; Wadhwa PD; Bajor DJ; Creger RJ; Xu Z; Cooper BW; Laughlin MJ; Gerson SL; Koc ON; Lazarus HM
Institution:	Department of Epidemiology and Biostatistics, Case Comprehensive Cancer Center, Cleveland, Ohio 44106, United States. pxf16@case.edu
Journal:	Contemp Clin Trials. 2008 Mar;29(2):157-64. Epub 2007 Jul 19.
Abstract Link:	http://www.medifocus.com/abstracts.php?gid=HM009&ID=17707140

216.

High-dose chemotherapy and autologous hematopoietic progenitor cell transplantation for non-Hodgkin's lymphoma in patients >65 years of age.

Authors:	Hosing C; Saliba RM; Okoroji GJ; Popat U; Couriel D; Ali T; De Padua Silva L; Kebriaei P; Alousi A; De Lima M; Qazilbash M; Anderlini P; Giralt S; Champlin RE; Khouri I
Institution:	Department of Stem Cell Transplantation and Cellular Therapy, The University of Texas M. D. Anderson Cancer Center, Houston, TX 77030, USA. cmhosing@mdanderson.org
Journal:	Ann Oncol. 2008 Jun;19(6):1166-71. Epub 2008 Feb 13.
Abstract Link:	http://www.medifocus.com/abstracts.php?gid=HM009&ID=18272911

Go to http://www.medifocus.com/links/HM009/0212 for direct online access to the above Abstract Links.

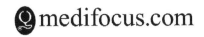
217.

High-dose chemotherapy with autologous stem cell support in first-line treatment of aggressive non-Hodgkin lymphoma - results of a comprehensive meta-analysis.

Authors:	Greb A; Bohlius J; Trelle S; Schiefer D; De Souza CA; Gisselbrecht C; Intragumtornchai T; Kaiser U; Kluin-Nelemans HC; Martelli M; Milpied NJ; Santini G; Verdonck LF; Vitolo U; Schwarzer G; Engert A
Institution:	Department of Internal Medicine I, University of Cologne, Cologne, Germany.
Journal:	Cancer Treat Rev. 2007 Jun;33(4):338-46. Epub 2007 Apr 2.
Abstract Link:	http://www.medifocus.com/abstracts.php?gid=HM009&ID=17400393

218.

Obesity in survivors of childhood acute lymphoblastic leukemia and lymphoma.

Authors:	Razzouk BI; Rose SR; Hongeng S; Wallace D; Smeltzer MP; Zacher M; Pui CH; Hudson MM
Institution:	Department of Hematology-Oncology, St Jude Children's Research Hospital and the University of Tennessee Health Science Center, Memphis, TN 38105-2794, USA. bassem.razzouk@stjude.org
Journal:	J Clin Oncol. 2007 Apr 1;25(10):1183-9.
Abstract Link:	http://www.medifocus.com/abstracts.php?gid=HM009&ID=17401007

219.

Diabetes and risk of non-Hodgkin lymphoma: a case-control study.

Authors:	Scotti L; Tavani A; Bosetti C; Maso LD; Talamini R; Montella M; Franceschi S; La Vecchia C
Institution:	Istituto di Ricerche Farmacologiche Mario Negri, Milan, Italy.
Journal:	Tumori. 2007 Jan-Feb;93(1):1-3.
Abstract Link:	http://www.medifocus.com/abstracts.php?gid=HM009&ID=17455863

Go to http://www.medifocus.com/links/HM009/0212 for direct online access to the above Abstract Links.

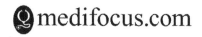

Radioimmunotherapy Articles

220.

B-cell non-Hodgkin lymphoma: PET/CT evaluation after 90Y-ibritumomab tiuxetan radioimmunotherapy--initial experience.

Authors: Ulaner GA; Colletti PM; Conti PS

Institution: Department of Radiology, University of Southern California, 1200 N State St, GNH 3550, Los Angeles, CA 90033, USA. ulaner@usc.edu

Journal: Radiology. 2008 Mar;246(3):895-902. Epub 2008 Feb 7.

Abstract Link: http://www.medifocus.com/abstracts.php?gid=HM009&ID=18258810

221.

Current status and future perspectives for yttrium-90 ((90)Y)-ibritumomab tiuxetan in stem cell transplantation for non-Hodgkin's lymphoma.

Authors: Gisselbrecht C; Bethge W; Duarte RF; Gianni AM; Glass B; Haioun C; Martinelli G; Nagler A; Pettengell R; Sureda A; Tilly H; Wilson K

Institution: Institut d'Hematologie, Hopital Saint-Louis, Paris, France. christian.gisselbrecht@sls.ap-hop-paris.fr

Journal: Bone Marrow Transplant. 2007 Dec;40(11):1007-17. Epub 2007 Oct 8.

Abstract Link: http://www.medifocus.com/abstracts.php?gid=HM009&ID=17922042

222.

Radioimmunotherapy as a therapeutic option for Non-Hodgkin's lymphoma.

Author: Macklis RM

Institution: Cleveland Clinic Lerner College of Medicine and Department of Radiation Oncology, Cleveland Clinic Foundation, Cleveland, OH 44195, USA. macklir@ccf.org

Journal: Semin Radiat Oncol. 2007 Jul;17(3):176-83.

Abstract Link: http://www.medifocus.com/abstracts.php?gid=HM009&ID=17591564

Go to http://www.medifocus.com/links/HM009/0212 for direct online access to the above Abstract Links.

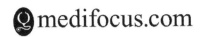

223.

Iodine 131 tositumomab in the treatment of non-Hodgkin's lymphoma.

Authors: Smith S; Sweetenham JW

Institution: Cleveland Clinic Foundation, Department of Hematology/Oncology, Taussig Cancer Center, 9500 Euclid Avenue R35, Cleveland, OH 44195, USA. smiths11@ccf.org

Journal: Future Oncol. 2007 Jun;3(3):255-62.

Abstract Link: http://www.medifocus.com/abstracts.php?gid=HM009&ID=17547519

224.

Radioimmunotherapy in the treatment of non-Hodgkin's lymphoma.

Author: Whelton S

Institution: Rush University Medical Center, Division of Hematology, Chicago, Illinois, USA.

Journal: Nurse Pract. 2007 Dec;32(12):35-8.

Abstract Link: **ABSTRACT NOT AVAILABLE**

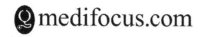

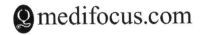

NOTES

Use this page for taking notes as you review your Guidebook

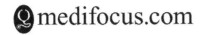 medifocus.com

4 - Centers of Research

This section of your *MediFocus Guidebook* is a unique directory of doctors, researchers, medical centers, and research institutions with specialized research interest, and in many cases, clinical expertise in the management of this specific medical condition. The *Centers of Research* directory is a valuable resource for quickly identifying and locating leading medical authorities and medical institutions within the United States and other countries that are considered to be at the forefront in clinical research and treatment of this disorder.

Use the *Centers of Research* directory to contact, consult, or network with leading experts in the field and to locate a hospital or medical center that can help you.

The following information is provided in the *Centers of Research* directory:

- **Geographic Location**

  - United States: the information is divided by individual states listed in alphabetical order. Not all states may be included.

  - Other Countries: information is presented for select countries worldwide listed in alphabetical order. Not all countries may be included.

- **Names of Authors**

  - Select names of individual authors (doctors, researchers, or other health-care professionals) with specialized research interest, and in many cases, clinical expertise in the management of this specific medical condition, who have recently published articles in leading medical journals about the condition.

  - E-mail addresses for individual authors, if listed on their specific publications, is also provided.

- **Institutional Affiliations**

  - Next to each individual author's name is their **institutional affiliation** (hospital, medical center, or research institution) where the study was conducted as listed in their publication(s).

- In many cases, information about the specific **department** within the medical institution where the individual author was located at the time the study was conducted is also provided.

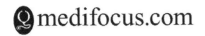

Centers of Research

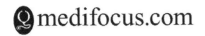

United States

AL - Alabama

Name of Author	Institutional Affiliation
Forero A	Department of Medicine, Division of Hematology/Oncology, University of Alabama at Birmingham Comprehensive Cancer Center, Birmingham, AL, USA.
Shah J	Department of Medicine, Division of Hematology/Oncology, University of Alabama at Birmingham Comprehensive Cancer Center, Birmingham, AL, USA.

AZ - Arizona

Name of Author	Institutional Affiliation
Fisher RI	Arizona Cancer Center, Tucson, AZ, USA. dmahadevan@azcc.arizona.edu
Mahadevan D	Arizona Cancer Center, Tucson, AZ, USA. dmahadevan@azcc.arizona.edu

CA - California

Name of Author	Institutional Affiliation
Advani R	Division of Oncology, Stanford University Medical Center, 875 Blake Wilbur Dr, Stanford, CA 94305, USA. radvani@stanford.edu
Bernstein L	Department of Population Sciences, Beckman Research Institute, City of Hope, 1500 East Duarte Road, Duarte, CA 91010, USA. yalu@coh.org
Chao MP	Institute for Stem Cell Biology and Regenerative Medicine, Stanford Cancer Center, and Ludwig Center at Stanford, Stanford, CA, USA. mpchao@stanford.edu

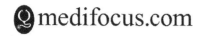

Conti PS	Department of Radiology, University of Southern California, 1200 N State St, GNH 3550, Los Angeles, CA 90033, USA. ulaner@usc.edu
Drachman JG	Division of Oncology, Stanford University Medical Center, 875 Blake Wilbur Dr, Stanford, CA 94305, USA. radvani@stanford.edu
Ebens A	Research and Early Development, Genentech, South San Francisco, CA 94080, USA. polson@gene.com
Forman SJ	Division of Hematology and Hematopoietic Cell Transplantation, City of Hope Comprehensive Cancer Center, Duarte, CA 91010, USA. akrishnan@coh.org
Holly EA	Division of Endocrinology, Clinical Nutrition, and Vascular Medicine, Department of Internal Medicine, University of California Davis, Sacramento, CA, USA.
Krishnan A	Division of Hematology and Hematopoietic Cell Transplantation, City of Hope Comprehensive Cancer Center, Duarte, CA 91010, USA. akrishnan@coh.org
Lee JS	Division of Endocrinology, Clinical Nutrition, and Vascular Medicine, Department of Internal Medicine, University of California Davis, Sacramento, CA, USA.
Lu Y	Department of Population Sciences, Beckman Research Institute, City of Hope, 1500 East Duarte Road, Duarte, CA 91010, USA. yalu@coh.org
Polson AG	Research and Early Development, Genentech, South San Francisco, CA 94080, USA. polson@gene.com
Rubenstein JL	Division of Hematology/Oncology, and the Department of Epidemiology and Biostatistics, University of California, San Francisco, San Francisco, CA 94143, USA. jamesr@medicine.ucsf.edu
Saven A	Division of Hematology/Oncology, Scripps Clinic, 10666 N. Torrey Pines Road, M/S 217 La Jolla, CA 92037, USA. sigal.darren@scrippshealth.org
Shuman M	Division of Hematology/Oncology, and the Department of Epidemiology and Biostatistics, University of California, San Francisco, San Francisco, CA 94143, USA. jamesr@medicine.ucsf.edu

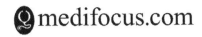

Sigal DS	Division of Hematology/Oncology, Scripps Clinic, 10666 N. Torrey Pines Road, M/S 217 La Jolla, CA 92037, USA. sigal.darren@scrippshealth.org
Skibola CF	Division of Environmental Health Sciences, School of Public Health, 140 Earl Warren Hall, University of California, Berkeley, CA 94720-7360, USA. chrisfs@berkeley.edu
Smith AH	Center for Occupational and Environmental Health, School of Public Health, 216 Earl Warren Hall, University of California, Berkeley, CA 94720-7360, USA. martynts@berkeley.edu
Smith MT	Center for Occupational and Environmental Health, School of Public Health, 216 Earl Warren Hall, University of California, Berkeley, CA 94720-7360, USA. martynts@berkeley.edu
Ulaner GA	Department of Radiology, University of Southern California, 1200 N State St, GNH 3550, Los Angeles, CA 90033, USA. ulaner@usc.edu
Weissman IL	Institute for Stem Cell Biology and Regenerative Medicine, Stanford Cancer Center, and Ludwig Center at Stanford, Stanford, CA, USA. mpchao@stanford.edu

CO - Colorado

Name of Author	Institutional Affiliation
Gore L	Center for Cancer and Blood Disorders, The Children's Hospital, The University of Colorado Cancer Center, Denver, 80045, USA. lia.gore@ucdenver.edu
Trippett TM	Center for Cancer and Blood Disorders, The Children's Hospital, The University of Colorado Cancer Center, Denver, 80045, USA. lia.gore@ucdenver.edu

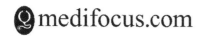

CT - Connecticut

Name of Author	Institutional Affiliation
Aziz NM	Department of Human Development and Family Studies, University of Connecticut, 348 Mansfield Rd, Unit 2058, Storrs, CT 06269, USA. Keith.M.Bellizzi@Uconn.edu
Bellizzi KM	Department of Human Development and Family Studies, University of Connecticut, 348 Mansfield Rd, Unit 2058, Storrs, CT 06269, USA. Keith.M.Bellizzi@Uconn.edu

DC - Washington D.C.

Name of Author	Institutional Affiliation
Cheson BD	Georgetown University Hospital, Lombardi Comprehensive Cancer Center, 3800 Reservoir RD, NW, Washington, DC 20007, USA.
Diehl V	Division of Hematology/Oncology, Georgetown University Hospital, Washington, DC, USA. bdc4@georgetown.edu
Rummel M	Division of Hematology-Oncology, Georgetown University Hospital, Lombardi Comprehensive Cancer Center, Washington, DC 20007, USA. bdc4@georgetown.edu
Ujjani C	Georgetown University Hospital, Lombardi Comprehensive Cancer Center, 3800 Reservoir RD, NW, Washington, DC 20007, USA.

FL - Florida

Name of Author	Institutional Affiliation
Bello C	H Lee Moffitt Cancer, 12901 Magnolia Drive, FOB3, Tampa, FL 33612, USA. celeste.bello@moffitt.org
Pinilla-Ibarz J	H Lee Moffitt Cancer, 12901 Magnolia Drive, FOB3, Tampa, FL 33612, USA. celeste.bello@moffitt.org

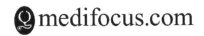 **medifocus.com**

IA - Iowa

Name of Author	**Institutional Affiliation**
Halwani AS	Department of Medicine, University of Iowa College of Medicine, Holden Comprehensive Cancer Center, 200 Hawkins Drive, Iowa City, IA 52242, USA.
Leonard JP	University of Iowa Hospitals and Clinics, Iowa City, IA, USA.
Link BK	University of Iowa Hospitals and Clinics, Iowa City, IA, USA.

IL - Illinois

Name of Author	**Institutional Affiliation**
Ahmed S	Division of Hematology/Oncology, Northwestern University Feinberg School of Medicine, Chicago, IL, USA.
Chiu BC	Department of Preventive Medicine, Feinberg School of Medicine, Northwestern University, 680 North Lake Shore Drive, Suite 1102, Chicago, IL, 60611-4402, USA.
Evens AM	Division of Hematology/Oncology, Northwestern University Feinberg School of Medicine, Chicago, IL, USA.
Hari PN	University of Chicago Medical Center, Chicago, Illinois, USA. kvbesien@uchicago.edu
Horning SJ	Feinberg School of Medicine-Northwestern University, Chicago, IL 60611, USA. t-kuzel@northwestern.edu
Kuzel TM	Feinberg School of Medicine-Northwestern University, Chicago, IL 60611, USA. t-kuzel@northwestern.edu
Nabhan C	Division of Hematology and Medical Oncology and Hematology and Oncology Fellowship Program, Advocate Lutheran General Hospital, Park Ridge, IL 60068, USA. Illinois. cnabhan@oncmed.net
Poire X	Department of Medicine, University of Chicago Medical Center, Chicago, IL 60637, USA.
Smith SM	Department of Medicine, University of Chicago Medical Center, Chicago, IL 60637, USA.

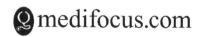 medifocus.com

Venugopal P	Division of Hematology and Medical Oncology and Hematology and Oncology Fellowship Program, Advocate Lutheran General Hospital, Park Ridge, IL 60068, USA. Illinois. cnabhan@oncmed.net
Weisenburger DD	Department of Preventive Medicine, Feinberg School of Medicine, Northwestern University, 680 North Lake Shore Drive, Suite 1102, Chicago, IL, 60611-4402, USA.
Whelton S	Rush University Medical Center, Division of Hematology, Chicago, Illinois, USA.
van Besien K	University of Chicago Medical Center, Chicago, Illinois, USA. kvbesien@uchicago.edu

IN - Indiana

Name of Author	**Institutional Affiliation**
Calandra G	Indiana Blood & Marrow Transplantation, Indianapolis, IN 46107, USA. mdugan@ibmtindy.com
Dugan MJ	Indiana Blood & Marrow Transplantation, Indianapolis, IN 46107, USA. mdugan@ibmtindy.com
Farag SS	Department of Medicine, Indiana University School of Medicine, Indianapolis, Indiana 46202, USA.
Srivastava S	Department of Medicine, Indiana University School of Medicine, Indianapolis, Indiana 46202, USA.

LA - Louisiana

Name of Author	**Institutional Affiliation**
Collins-Burow B	Tulane University School of Medicine, Division of Hematology-Medical Oncology, Tulane Cancer Center, 1430 Tulane Avenue, SL-78, New Orleans, LA 70112, USA. bcollin1@tulane.edu
Santos ES	Tulane University School of Medicine, Division of Hematology-Medical Oncology, Tulane Cancer Center, 1430 Tulane Avenue, SL-78, New Orleans, LA 70112, USA. bcollin1@tulane.edu

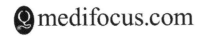medifocus.com

MA - Massachussetts

Name of Author	Institutional Affiliation
Ballen KK	Division of Hematology/Oncology, Department of Medicine, Massachusetts General Hospital, Boston, MA 02114, USA.
Batchelor T	Massachusetts General Hospital and Harvard Medical School, Department of Neurology, Boston, MA 02114, USA. egerstner@partners.org
Batchelor TT	Division of Hematology and Oncology, Massachusetts General Hospital Cancer Center and Harvard Medical School, Boston, MA, USA. egerstner@partners.org
Chen YB	Department of Hematology/Oncology, Massachusetts General Hospital, Boston, Massachusetts 02114, USA.
Claus EB	Center for Neuro-Oncology, Dana-Farber/Brigham and Women's Cancer Center, 44 Binney St, Boston, MA 02115, USA. anorden@partners.org
Gerstner E	Massachusetts General Hospital and Harvard Medical School, Department of Neurology, Boston, MA 02114, USA. egerstner@partners.org
Gerstner ER	Division of Hematology and Oncology, Massachusetts General Hospital Cancer Center and Harvard Medical School, Boston, MA, USA. egerstner@partners.org
Kemp S	Department of Oral and Maxillofacial Pathology, Boston University School of Dental Medicine, Boston, MA 02118, USA. skemp@bu.edu
Martin NE	Harvard Radiation Oncology Program, Brigham and Women's Hospital/Dana-Farber Cancer Institute, Boston, MA 02115, USA.
Ng AK	Harvard Radiation Oncology Program, Brigham and Women's Hospital/Dana-Farber Cancer Institute, Boston, MA 02115, USA.
Norden AD	Center for Neuro-Oncology, Dana-Farber/Brigham and Women's Cancer Center, 44 Binney St, Boston, MA 02115, USA. anorden@partners.org

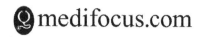

O'Hara C	Department of Oral and Maxillofacial Pathology, Boston University School of Dental Medicine, Boston, MA 02118, USA. skemp@bu.edu
Silva M	Department of Pharmacy Practice, Massachusetts College of Pharmacy and Health Sciences, Worcester, Massachusetts 01608, USA. michael.steinberg@mcphs.edu
Steinberg M	Department of Pharmacy Practice, Massachusetts College of Pharmacy and Health Sciences, Worcester, Massachusetts 01608, USA. michael.steinberg@mcphs.edu
Ulrickson M	Department of Hematology/Oncology, Massachusetts General Hospital, Boston, Massachusetts 02114, USA.
Yusuf RZ	Division of Hematology/Oncology, Department of Medicine, Massachusetts General Hospital, Boston, MA 02114, USA.

MD - Maryland

Name of Author	Institutional Affiliation
6Schaefer NG	Division of Nuclear Medicine, Russell H. Morgan Department of Radiology and Radiological Sciences, Sidney Kimmell Cancer Center, Johns Hopkins University School of Medicine, Baltimore, Maryland 21287-0817, USA.
Anderson LA	Viral Epidemiology Branch, Division of Cancer Epidemiology and Genetics, National Cancer Institute, NIH, Bethesda, MD 20892, USA. l.anderson@qub.ac.uk
Chen, Xing-Zhen	Division of Nuclear Medicine, Russell H. Morgan Department of Radiology and Radiological Sciences, Sidney Kimmell Cancer Center, Johns Hopkins University School of Medicine, Baltimore, Maryland 21287-0817, USA.
Engels EA	Division of Cancer Epidemiology and Genetics, National Cancer Institute, NIH, Department of Health and Human Services, 6120 Executive Boulevard, EPS 7076, Rockville, MD 20852, USA. engelse@exchange.nih.gov
Hartge P	National Cancer Institute, NIH, Department of Health and Human Services, Rockville, MD 20892, USA. hartge@nih.gov

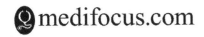

Landgren O	Viral Epidemiology Branch, Division of Cancer Epidemiology and Genetics, National Cancer Institute, NIH, Bethesda, MD 20892, USA. l.anderson@qub.ac.uk
Smith MT	National Cancer Institute, NIH, Department of Health and Human Services, Rockville, MD 20892, USA. hartge@nih.gov

MN - Minnesota

Name of Author	Institutional Affiliation
Bachanova V	Blood and Marrow, Transplant Program, University of Minnesota, Minneapolis, MN 55455, USA. bach0173@umn.edu
Cerhan JR	Department of Health Sciences Research, College of Medicine, Mayo Clinic, Rochester, MN 55905, USA.
Geyer SM	Department of Health Sciences Research, College of Medicine, Mayo Clinic, Rochester, MN 55905, USA.
Habermann TM	Division of Hematology, Department of Medicine, Mayo Clinic College of Medicine and Mayo Foundation, Rochester, MN 55905, USA. Witzig@mayo.edu
Holtan SG	Department of Medicine, Mayo Clinic College of Medicine, Rochester, MN 55905, USA.
Laack NN	Department of Radiation Oncology, Mayo Clinic and Mayo Foundation, Rochester, Minnesota 55905, USA.
Leukemia GB	University of Minnesota. Minneapolis, MN. USA.
Markovic SN	Department of Medicine, Mayo Clinic College of Medicine, Rochester, MN 55905, USA.
Miller JS	Blood and Marrow, Transplant Program, University of Minnesota, Minneapolis, MN 55455, USA. bach0173@umn.edu
Pajon ER Jr	Department of Radiation Oncology, Mayo Clinic and Mayo Foundation, Rochester, Minnesota 55905, USA.
Peterson BA	University of Minnesota. Minneapolis, MN. USA.
Vose JM	Mayo Clinic, Rochester, MN 55905, USA. witzig@mayo.edu

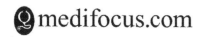

| Witzig TE | Mayo Clinic, Rochester, MN 55905, USA. witzig@mayo.edu |

MO - Missouri

Name of Author	Institutional Affiliation
Calandra G	Washington University School of Medicine, St Louis, MO, USA. jdipersi@im.wustl.edu
DiPersio JF	Washington University School of Medicine, St Louis, MO, USA. jdipersi@im.wustl.edu

NC - North Carolina

Name of Author	Institutional Affiliation
Ganz PA	Duke University Medical Center, DUMC 2732, Durham, NC 27710, USA. sophia.smith@duke.edu
Smith SK	Sheps Center for Health Services Research, University of North Carolina, Chapel Hill, NC, USA. sophia_smith@unc.edu
Zebrack BJ	Sheps Center for Health Services Research, University of North Carolina, Chapel Hill, NC, USA. sophia_smith@unc.edu

NJ - New Jersey

Name of Author	Institutional Affiliation
Bertino JR	Department of Medicine, University of Medicine and Dentistry, Robert Wood Johnson Medical School, and The Cancer Institute of New Jersey, New Brusnwick, NJ 08901, USA.
Levitt MJ	Department of Medicine, University of Medicine and Dentistry, Robert Wood Johnson Medical School, and The Cancer Institute of New Jersey, New Brusnwick, NJ 08901, USA.

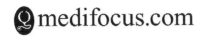

NV - Nevada

Name of Author	Institutional Affiliation
Dang NH	Department of Hematologic Malignancies, Nevada Cancer Institute, Las Vegas, NV 89135, USA. ndang@nvcancer.org
Pro B	Department of Hematologic Malignancies, Nevada Cancer Institute, Las Vegas, NV 89135, USA. ndang@nvcancer.org

NY - New York

Name of Author	Institutional Affiliation
Abrey LE	Department of Medicine, Memorial Sloan-Kettering Cancer Center, New York, NY 10065, USA.
Bhat S	Roswell Park Cancer Institute, Elm and Carlton Streets, Buffalo, NY 14263, USA.
Cai S	Department of Surgery, The State University of New York at Buffalo, Buffalo, NY, USA.
Cairo MS	Department of Pediatrics, Columbia University, New York, NY 10032, USA.
Chanan-Khan AA	Roswell Park Cancer Institute, Buffalo, NY, USA. asher.chanan-khan@roswellpark.org
Cheson BD	James P. Wilmot Cancer Center, University of Rochester, 601 Elmwood Ave, Box 704, Rochester, NY, 14642, USA. Jonathan_Friedberg@URMC.Rochester.edu
Czuczman MS	Department of Pharmacy, Roswell Park Cancer Institute, Elm and Carlton Streets, Buffalo, NY 14263, USA. angie.elefante@roswellpark.org
Ekenel M	Department of Neurology, Memorial Sloan-Kettering Cancer Center, New York, New York 10065, USA.
Elefante A	Department of Pharmacy, Roswell Park Cancer Institute, Elm and Carlton Streets, Buffalo, NY 14263, USA. angie.elefante@roswellpark.org
Engel LS	Department of Epidemiology, Memorial Sloan-Kettering Cancer Center, Epidemiology Service, 307 E. 63rd St., 3rd Floor, New York, NY 10021, USA. engell@mskcc.org

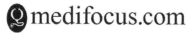

Forman SJ	Department of Medical Oncology, NYU Medical Center, New York, USA.
Friedberg J	James P. Wilmot Cancer Center, and Department of Medicine, University of Rochester, Rochester, NY, USA.
Friedberg JW	James P. Wilmot Cancer Center, University of Rochester, 601 Elmwood Ave, Box 704, Rochester, NY, 14642, USA. Jonathan_Friedberg@URMC.Rochester.edu
Graber JJ	Department of Neurology, Memorial Sloan-Kettering Cancer Center, New York, New York, USA.
Habermann TM	Our Lady of Mercy Cancer Center, New York Medical College, Bronx, NY, USA.
Hochberg J	Department of Pediatrics, Columbia University, New York, NY 10032, USA.
Horwitz SM	Memorial Sloan Kettering Cancer Center, New York, New York 10021, USA. horwitzs@mskcc.org
Leonard JP	Center for Lymphoma and Myeloma, Division of Hematology/Oncology, Weill Medical College of Cornell University and New York Presbyterian Hospital, New York, NY 10021, USA.
Martin P	Center for Lymphoma and Myeloma, Division of Hematology and Medical Oncology, Weill Medical College of Cornell University and New York Presbyterian Hospital, New York, NY 10021, USA.
Mones JV	Center for Lymphoma and Myeloma, Division of Hematology/Oncology, Weill Medical College of Cornell University and New York Presbyterian Hospital, New York, NY 10021, USA.
Morris PG	Department of Medicine, Memorial Sloan-Kettering Cancer Center, New York, NY 10065, USA.
O'Connor OA	NYU Cancer Institute, School of Medicine, NYU Langone Medical Center, New York, New York 10016, USA.
Omuro A	Department of Neurology, Memorial Sloan-Kettering Cancer Center, New York, New York, USA.
Rajput A	Department of Surgery, The State University of New York at Buffalo, Buffalo, NY, USA.

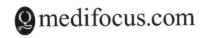

Reeder CB	Roswell Park Cancer Institute, Buffalo, NY 14263, USA. myron.czuczman@roswellpark.org
Rothman N	Department of Epidemiology, Memorial Sloan-Kettering Cancer Center, Epidemiology Service, 307 E. 63rd St., 3rd Floor, New York, NY 10021, USA. engell@mskcc.org
Sawas A	NYU Cancer Institute, School of Medicine, NYU Langone Medical Center, New York, New York 10016, USA.
Sousou T	James P. Wilmot Cancer Center, and Department of Medicine, University of Rochester, Rochester, NY, USA.
Teta MJ	Exponent, Inc., Health Sciences Practice, New York, New York, USA. jteta@exponent.com
Wagner ME	Exponent, Inc., Health Sciences Practice, New York, New York, USA. jteta@exponent.com
Wiernik PH	Our Lady of Mercy Cancer Center, New York Medical College, Bronx, NY, USA.
Zain J	Department of Medical Oncology, NYU Medical Center, New York, USA.
Zelenetz A	Department of Medicine, Division of Hematologic Oncology, Memorial Sloan Kettering Cancer Center, Lymphoma Service, New York, NY 10032, USA. oo2130@columbia.edu

OH - Ohio

Name of Author	Institutional Affiliation
Bolwell BJ	Taussig Cancer Institute, Cleveland Clinic, OH 44195, USA. deanr@ccf.org
Caimi PF	Department of Medicine, Case Comprehensive Cancer Center, University Hospitals Case Medical Center, Case Western Reserve University, Cleveland, Ohio 44106, USA.
Cairo MS	Division of Bone Marrow Transplant and Immune Deficiency, Cincinnati Children's Hospital Medical Center, Cincinnati, Ohio, USA. Richard.Harris@CCHMC.org
Dean RM	Taussig Cancer Institute, Cleveland Clinic, OH 44195, USA. deanr@ccf.org

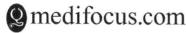

Devine SM	Hematology and Oncology, Arthur G James Comprehensive Cancer Center, The Ohio State University, Columbus, Ohio 43210, USA. mehdi.hamadani@gmail.com
Eapen M	Department of Pediatrics, Nationwide Children's Hospital, Ohio State University, Columbus, Ohio 43205, USA. thomas.gross@nationwidechildrens.org
Fu P	Department of Epidemiology and Biostatistics, Case Comprehensive Cancer Center, Cleveland, Ohio 44106, United States. pxf16@case.edu
Gross TG	Department of Pediatrics, Nationwide Children's Hospital, Ohio State University, Columbus, Ohio 43205, USA. thomas.gross@nationwidechildrens.org
Hamadani M	Hematology and Oncology, Arthur G James Comprehensive Cancer Center, The Ohio State University, Columbus, Ohio 43210, USA. mehdi.hamadani@gmail.com
Harris RE	Division of Bone Marrow Transplant and Immune Deficiency, Cincinnati Children's Hospital Medical Center, Cincinnati, Ohio, USA. Richard.Harris@CCHMC.org
Lazarus HM	Department of Epidemiology and Biostatistics, Case Comprehensive Cancer Center, Cleveland, Ohio 44106, United States. pxf16@case.edu
Macklis RM	Cleveland Clinic Lerner College of Medicine and Department of Radiation Oncology, Cleveland Clinic Foundation, Cleveland, OH 44195, USA. macklir@ccf.org
Smith S	Cleveland Clinic Foundation, Department of Hematology/Oncology, Taussig Cancer Center, 9500 Euclid Avenue R35, Cleveland, OH 44195, USA. smiths11@ccf.org
Sweetenham JW	Cleveland Clinic Foundation, Department of Hematology/Oncology, Taussig Cancer Center, 9500 Euclid Avenue R35, Cleveland, OH 44195, USA. smiths11@ccf.org

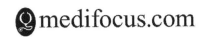

PA - Pennsylvania

Name of Author	Institutional Affiliation
Beckjord EB	Department of Psychiatry, University of Pittsburgh, Pennsylvania, USA. beckjorde@upmc.edu
Rowland JH	Department of Psychiatry, University of Pittsburgh, Pennsylvania, USA. beckjorde@upmc.edu

RI - Rhode Island

Name of Author	Institutional Affiliation
Castillo J	Brown University Warren Alpert Medical School, The Miriam Hospital, Division of Hematology and Oncology, 164 Summit Avenue, Providence, RI 02906, USA.
Mega AE	Department of Hematology/Oncology, The Miriam Hospital, 164 Summit Avenue, Providence, RI 02906, USA. jreagan@lifespan.org
Milani C	Brown University Warren Alpert Medical School, The Miriam Hospital, Division of Hematology and Oncology, 164 Summit Avenue, Providence, RI 02906, USA.
Reagan JL	Department of Hematology/Oncology, The Miriam Hospital, 164 Summit Avenue, Providence, RI 02906, USA. jreagan@lifespan.org

TN - Tennessee

Name of Author	Institutional Affiliation
Hudson MM	Department of Oncology, St Jude Children's Research Hospital, University of Tennessee, Memphis, TN, USA. John.Sandlund@stjude.org
Razzouk BI	Department of Hematology-Oncology, St Jude Children's Research Hospital and the University of Tennessee Health Science Center, Memphis, TN 38105-2794, USA. bassem.razzouk@stjude.org
Sandlund JT	Department of Oncology, St Jude Children's Research Hospital, University of Tennessee, Memphis, TN, USA. John.Sandlund@stjude.org

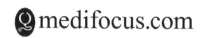

TX - Texas

Name of Author	Institutional Affiliation
Berrios-Rivera JP	Division of Epidemiology, University of Texas School of Public Health, Houston, Texas 77030, USA.
Beveridge R	Blood and Marrow Transplant Network, US Oncology Research, Inc, The Woodlands, TX, USA. robert.rifkin@usoncology.com
Cabanillas ME	Department of Leukemia, The University of Texas M.D. Anderson Cancer Center, Houston, TX, USA. mcabani@mdanderson.org
Champlin RE	Department of Stem Cell Transplantation and Cellular Therapy, The University of Texas MD Anderson Cancer Center, Houston, TX 77030, USA.
Czuczman MS	MD Anderson Cancer Center, 1515 Holcombe Boulevard, Houston, TX 77030-4009, USA. ayounes@mdanderson.org
Du XL	Department of Leukemia, The University of Texas M.D. Anderson Cancer Center, Houston, TX, USA. mcabani@mdanderson.org
Fanale MA	Department of Lymphoma/Myeloma, The University of Texas M.D. Anderson Cancer Center, Houston, Texas, USA. mfanale@mdanderson.org
Fayad LE	Department of Lymphoma and Myeloma, University of Texas MD Anderson Cancer Center, Houston, Texas, USA.
Hagemeister FB	Department of Lymphoma/Myeloma, M. D. Anderson Cancer Center, Houston, TX 77030, USA. fhagemei@mdanderson.org
Hosing C	Department of Stem Cell Transplantation and Cellular Therapy, The University of Texas MD Anderson Cancer Center, Houston, TX 77030, USA.
Khouri I	Department of Stem Cell Transplantation and Cellular Therapy, The University of Texas M. D. Anderson Cancer Center, Houston, TX 77030, USA. cmhosing@mdanderson.org
Krance R	Texas Children's Cancer Center, Houston, TX 77030, USA. fvokur@txccc.org

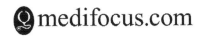

Lee ST | The University of Texas M. D. Anderson Cancer Center, Department of Lymphoma and Myeloma, Division of Cancer Medicine, 1515 Holcombe Blvd, Unit 903, Houston, TX, 77030 USA. stlee@mdanderson.org

Neelapu SS | The University of Texas M. D. Anderson Cancer Center, Department of Lymphoma and Myeloma, Division of Cancer Medicine, 1515 Holcombe Blvd, Unit 903, Houston, TX, 77030 USA. stlee@mdanderson.org

Okur FV | Texas Children's Cancer Center, Houston, TX 77030, USA. fvokur@txccc.org

Rifkin R | Blood and Marrow Transplant Network, US Oncology Research, Inc, The Woodlands, TX, USA. robert.rifkin@usoncology.com

Rodriguez MA | Lymphoma/Myeloma Department, The University of Texas M. D. Anderson Cancer Center, Houston, Texas 77030, USA. marodriguez@mdanderson.org

Srokowski TP | Department of Lymphoma and Myeloma, University of Texas MD Anderson Cancer Center, Houston, Texas, USA.

Winter JN | Lymphoma/Myeloma Department, The University of Texas M. D. Anderson Cancer Center, Houston, Texas 77030, USA. marodriguez@mdanderson.org

Younes A | MD Anderson Cancer Center, 1515 Holcombe Boulevard, Houston, TX 77030-4009, USA. ayounes@mdanderson.org

UT - Utah

Name of Author	Institutional Affiliation
Gaffney D	Huntsman Cancer Hospital, University of Utah, UT 84112-5560, USA. Jonathan.Tward@hci.utah.edu
Gaffney DK	Department of Radiation Oncology, Huntsman Cancer Hospital and the University of Utah, Salt Lake City, Utah 84112, USA.
Tward J	Huntsman Cancer Hospital, University of Utah, UT 84112-5560, USA. Jonathan.Tward@hci.utah.edu
Wendland MM	Department of Radiation Oncology, Huntsman Cancer Hospital and the University of Utah, Salt Lake City, Utah 84112, USA.

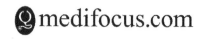

WA - Washington

Name of Author	Institutional Affiliation
Fefer A	Puget Sound Oncology Consortium, Seattle, WA, USA. jat@u.washington.edu
Gisselbrecht C	Fred Hutchinson Cancer Research Center, Division of Oncology, University of Washington, Seattle, USA.
Maloney D	Fred Hutchinson Cancer Research Center, Division of Oncology, University of Washington, Seattle, USA.
Maloney DG	Fred Hutchinson Cancer Research Center, 1100 Fairview Ave N, MS D1-100, Seattle, WA 98109, USA.
Palanca-Wessels MC	Division of Hematology, Department of Medicine, Fred Hutchinson Cancer Research Center, University of Washington, 1100 Fairview Avenue N., Seattle, WA 98109, USA.
Press OW	Division of Hematology, Department of Medicine, Fred Hutchinson Cancer Research Center, University of Washington, 1100 Fairview Avenue N., Seattle, WA 98109, USA.
Rezvani AR	Fred Hutchinson Cancer Research Center, 1100 Fairview Ave N, MS D1-100, Seattle, WA 98109, USA.
Thompson JA	Puget Sound Oncology Consortium, Seattle, WA, USA. jat@u.washington.edu

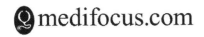

Centers of Research

Australia

Name of Author	Institutional Affiliation
Armstrong BK	Sydney Cancer Centre, Royal Prince Alfred Hospital, Missenden Road, Camperdown 2050, Sydney, New South Wales, Australia. brucea@health.usyd.edu.au
Bashford J	Department of Clinical Haematology and Bone Marrow Transplantation, Royal Melbourne Hospital and University of Melbourne, Melbourne, Australia. Andrew.grigg@mh.org.au
Cozen W	National Centre in HIV Epidemiology and Clinical Research, Level 2, 376 Victoria Street, Darlinghurst, NSW 2010, Australia. agrulich@nchecr.unsw.edu.au
Grigg AP	Department of Clinical Haematology and Bone Marrow Transplantation, Royal Melbourne Hospital and University of Melbourne, Melbourne, Australia. Andrew.grigg@mh.org.au
Grulich AE	National Centre in HIV Epidemiology and Clinical Research, Level 2, 376 Victoria Street, Darlinghurst, NSW 2010, Australia. agrulich@nchecr.unsw.edu.au
Kricker A	Sydney Cancer Centre, Royal Prince Alfred Hospital, Missenden Road, Camperdown 2050, Sydney, New South Wales, Australia. brucea@health.usyd.edu.au

Austria

Name of Author	Institutional Affiliation
Fridrik MA	Department Internal Medicine 3, Centre for Hematology and Medical Oncology, General Hospital Linz, Krankenhausstrasse 9, 4020, Linz, Austria. michael.fridrik@akh.linz.at

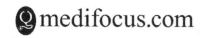

Greil R Department Internal Medicine 3, Centre for Hematology and Medical Oncology, General Hospital Linz, Krankenhausstrasse 9, 4020, Linz, Austria. michael.fridrik@akh.linz.at

Bosnia and Herzegovina

Name of Author | **Institutional Affiliation**

Hasic S
Clinic for Oncology, Hematology and Radiotherapy, Department of Hematology, University Clinical Center Tuzla, Tuzla, Bosnia and Herzegovina. samira.hasic@ukc.ba

Mazalovic E
Clinic for Oncology, Hematology and Radiotherapy, Department of Hematology, University Clinical Center Tuzla, Tuzla, Bosnia and Herzegovina. samira.hasic@ukc.ba

Canada

Name of Author | **Institutional Affiliation**

Al-Tourah AJ
Division of Medical Oncology, Fraser Valley and Vancouver Cancer Centers and the Department of Pathology and Biostatistics, British Columbia Cancer Agency and the University of British Columbia, Vancouver, BC, Canada. aaltoura@bccancer.bc.ca

Cheung MC
Cancer Care Ontario Program in Evidence-Based Care, McMaster University, Hamilton, Ont., Canada L8S 4L8. matthew.cheung@utoronto.ca <matthew.cheung@utoronto.ca>

Connors JM
Division of Medical Oncology, Fraser Valley and Vancouver Cancer Centers and the Department of Pathology and Biostatistics, British Columbia Cancer Agency and the University of British Columbia, Vancouver, BC, Canada. aaltoura@bccancer.bc.ca

Elphee EE
Malignant Hematology and Lymphoma Disease Site Group, Cancer Care Manitoba, Canada. erin.elphee@cancercare.mb.ca

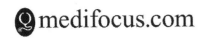

Gospodarowicz MK	Department of Radiation Oncology, University of Toronto, Princess Margaret Hospital, Toronto, Ontario, Canada. Richard.tsang@rmp.uhn.on.ca
Imrie KR	Cancer Care Ontario Program in Evidence-Based Care, McMaster University, Hamilton, Ont., Canada L8S 4L8. matthew.cheung@utoronto.ca <matthew.cheung@utoronto.ca>
Tsang RW	Department of Radiation Oncology, University of Toronto, Princess Margaret Hospital, Toronto, Ontario, Canada. Richard.tsang@rmp.uhn.on.ca

China

Name of Author	**Institutional Affiliation**
Cao J	Department of Medical Oncology, Fudan University Cancer Hospital, Shanghai, China.
Ghimire P	Department of Magnetic Resonance Imaging, Zhongnan Hospital, Wuhan University, 169 East Lake Road, Wuhan 430071, Hubei Province, China.
Jiang C	Department of Internal Medicine Oncology, Shandong Cancer Hospital, Shandong Academy of Medical Sciences, Jinan, Shandong 250117, China. zlysxgy@yahoo.com.cn
Kwong YL	Department of Medicine, University of Hong Kong, Hong Kong, China.
Lin T	State Key Laboratory of Oncology in South China, Department of Medical Oncology, Sun Yat-Sen University Cancer Center, 651 Dong Feng Road East, 510060, Guangzhou, Guangdong, People's Republic of China.
Liu L	Department of Hematology, Union Hospital, Tongji Medical College, Huazhong University of Science and Technology, Wuhan, China.
Liu X	Department of Medical Oncology, Fudan University Cancer Hospital, Shanghai, China.
Wang J	Department of Hematology, The Affiliated DrumTower Hospital of Nanjing University Medical School, 210008, Nanjing, People's Republic of China.

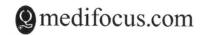
Yang XG	Department of Internal Medicine Oncology, Shandong Cancer Hospital, Shandong Academy of Medical Sciences, Jinan, Shandong 250117, China. zlysxgy@yahoo.com.cn
Yang Y	Department of Hematology, The Affiliated DrumTower Hospital of Nanjing University Medical School, 210008, Nanjing, People's Republic of China.
Zhai L	State Key Laboratory of Oncology in South China, Department of Medical Oncology, Sun Yat-Sen University Cancer Center, 651 Dong Feng Road East, 510060, Guangzhou, Guangdong, People's Republic of China.
Zhu L	Department of Magnetic Resonance Imaging, Zhongnan Hospital, Wuhan University, 169 East Lake Road, Wuhan 430071, Hubei Province, China.
Zou P	Department of Hematology, Union Hospital, Tongji Medical College, Huazhong University of Science and Technology, Wuhan, China.

Croatia

Name of Author	Institutional Affiliation
Aurer I	Division of Hematology, Department of Internal Medicine, University Hospital Center Zagreb, Kispaticeva 12, Zagreb, Croatia. aurer@mef.hr
Jaksic B	Department of Medicine, "Merkur" University Hospital, Zagreb, Croatia. delfaradic@kb.merkur.com
Radic-Kristo D	Department of Medicine, "Merkur" University Hospital, Zagreb, Croatia. delfaradic@kb.merkur.com
van der Maazen RW	Division of Hematology, Department of Internal Medicine, University Hospital Center Zagreb, Kispaticeva 12, Zagreb, Croatia. aurer@mef.hr

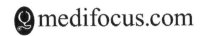

Czech Republic

Name of Author	Institutional Affiliation
Reinis M	Academy of Sciences of the Czech Republic, Institute of Molecular Genetics, Videnska 1083, Prague 4, CZ-14220, Czech Republic. reinis@img.cas.cz

Egypt

Name of Author	Institutional Affiliation
Azim HA	Department of Clinical Oncology, Cairo University Hospital, Cairo, Egypt.
Azim HA Jr	Department of Clinical Oncology, Cairo University Hospital, Cairo, Egypt.

France

Name of Author	Institutional Affiliation
Boffetta P	Gene-Environment Epidemiology Group, IARC, 150 cours Albert-Thomas, 69008 Lyon, France. boffetta@iarc.fr
Coiffier B	Departement d'Hematologie Clinique, Assistance Publique des Hopitaux de Paris, Hopital Saint-Louis, Institut Universitaire d'Hematologie, Paris. catherine.thieblemont@sls.aphp.fr
Desandes E	French National Registry of Childhood Solid Tumours, Universite Henri Poincare Nancy 1, Faculte de Medecine, 9, Avenue de la Foret de Haye, BP 184, 54505 Vandoeuvre-les-Nancy cedex, France.
Gisselbrecht C	Groupe d'Etude des Lymphomes de l'Adulte, GELA, 1 av C Vellefaux, Paris, France. mounier.n@chu-nice.fr
Goldenberg DM	Service des Maladies du Sang, Centre Hospitalier Regional, L'Universitaire de Lille, France.
Michallet AS	Hematologie, CH Lyon-Sud, 69495 Pierre-Benite, France. Anne-sophie.michallet@chu-lyon.fr

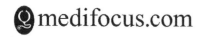

Morschhauser F	Service des Maladies du Sang, Centre Hospitalier Regional, L'Universitaire de Lille, France.
Mounier N	Groupe d'Etude des Lymphomes de l'Adulte, GELA, 1 av C Vellefaux, Paris, France. mounier.n@chu-nice.fr
Rainfray M	Medical Oncology Department, Institut Bergonie, 33076 Bordeaux Cedex, France. Soubeyran_p@bergonie.org
Soubeyran P	Medical Oncology Department, Institut Bergonie, 33076 Bordeaux Cedex, France. Soubeyran_p@bergonie.org
Thieblemont C	Departement d'Hematologie Clinique, Assistance Publique des Hopitaux de Paris, Hopital Saint-Louis, Institut Universitaire d'Hematologie, Paris. catherine.thieblemont@sls.aphp.fr
Wilson K	Institut d'Hematologie, Hopital Saint-Louis, Paris, France. christian.gisselbrecht@sls.ap-hop-paris.fr
de Vocht F	Gene-Environment Epidemiology Group, IARC, 150 cours Albert-Thomas, 69008 Lyon, France. boffetta@iarc.fr

Germany

Name of Author	Institutional Affiliation
Atta J	Department of Hematology, J. W. Goethe-University Hospital, Frankfurt, Germany. atta@em.uni-frankfurt.de
Boehme V	Department of Hematology and Stem Cell Transplantation, Asklepios Hospital St Georg, Hamburg, Germany.
Braun J	Rheumazentrum Ruhrgebiet, St. Josefs-Krankenhaus, Herne, Germany. kiltz@rheumazentrum-ruhrgbiet.de
Brenner H	Division of Clinical Epidemiology and Aging Research, German Cancer Research Center, Heidelberg, Germany.
Burkhardt B	NHL-BFM Study Center, Department of Pediatric Hematology and Oncology, Justus Liebig University, Giessen, Germany. birgit.burkhardt@paediat.med.uni-giessen.de
Busse A	Department of Medicine III, Charite, Campus Benjamin Franklin, Berlin, Germany.

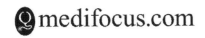

Cavalli F	Division of Clinical Neuro-oncology, Department of Neurology, University of Bonn, Bonn, Germany. Ulrich.Herrlinger@ukb.uni-bonn.de
Dierckx RA	Clinical Trials Center, University Medical Center, Elsasser Str. 2, D-79110 Freiburg, Germany. andreas.otte@uniklinik-freiburg.de
Dohler B	Department of Transplantation Immunology, Institute of Immunology, University of Heidelberg, Heidelberg, Germany. gerhard.opelz@med.uni-heidelberg.de
Duhrsen U	Department of Hematology, University Hospital Essen, University of Duisburg-Essen, Essen, Germany. ulrich.duehrsen@uk-essen.de
Engert A	Department of Internal Medicine I, University of Cologne, Cologne, Germany.
Fritsch K	Department of Hematology and Oncology, Freiburg University Medical Center, Freiburg, Germany.
Greb A	Department of Internal Medicine I, University of Cologne, Cologne, Germany.
Herrlinger U	Division of Clinical Neuro-oncology, Department of Neurology, University of Bonn, Bonn, Germany. Ulrich.Herrlinger@ukb.uni-bonn.de
Illerhaus G	Department of Hematology and Oncology, Freiburg University Medical Center, Freiburg, Germany.
Keilholz U	Department of Medicine III, Charite, Campus Benjamin Franklin, Berlin, Germany.
Kiewe P	Department of Hematology, Oncology, and Transfusion Medicine, Charite Universitatsmedizin Berlin, Campus Benjamin Franklin, Berlin, Germany. philipp.kiewe@charite.de
Kiltz U	Rheumazentrum Ruhrgebiet, St. Josefs-Krankenhaus, Herne, Germany. kiltz@rheumazentrum-ruhrgbiet.de
Korfel A	Department of Hematology, Oncology, and Transfusion Medicine, Charite Universitatsmedizin Berlin, Campus Benjamin Franklin, Berlin, Germany. philipp.kiewe@charite.de

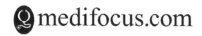

Loeffler M	Saarland University Medical School, Homburg, Germany. inmpfr@uniklinikum-saarland.de
Martin H	Department of Hematology, J. W. Goethe-University Hospital, Frankfurt, Germany. atta@em.uni-frankfurt.de
Muller S	Department of Hematology, University Hospital Essen, University of Duisburg-Essen, Essen, Germany. ulrich.duehrsen@uk-essen.de
Nowrousian MR	Department of Internal Medicine (Cancer Research), West German Cancer Center, University of Duisburg-Essen Medical School, Essen, Germany.
Opelz G	Department of Transplantation Immunology, Institute of Immunology, University of Heidelberg, Heidelberg, Germany. gerhard.opelz@med.uni-heidelberg.de
Otte A	Clinical Trials Center, University Medical Center, Elsasser Str. 2, D-79110 Freiburg, Germany. andreas.otte@uniklinik-freiburg.de
Pfreundschuh M	Innere Medizin I, Universitatskliniken des Saarlandes, Homburg, Germany.
Pulte D	Division of Clinical Epidemiology and Aging Research, German Cancer Research Center, Heidelberg, Germany.
Reiter A	NHL-BFM Study Center, Department of Pediatric Hematology and Oncology, Justus Liebig University, Giessen, Germany. birgit.burkhardt@paediat.med.uni-giessen.de
Rummel M	Department for Hematology and Medical Oncology, Justus-Liebig University Hospital, Giessen, Germany.
Schutt P	Department of Internal Medicine (Cancer Research), West German Cancer Center, University of Duisburg-Essen Medical School, Essen, Germany.
Trumper L	Hematology and Oncology, University Hospital Gottingen, Germany.
Zwick C	Innere Medizin I, Universitatskliniken des Saarlandes, Homburg, Germany.

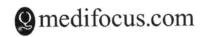

Greece

Name of Author	Institutional Affiliation
Antonopoulos CN	Department of Hygiene, Epidemiology and Medical Statistics, Athens University Medical School, Athens, Greece.
Falagas ME	Alfa Institute of Biomedical Sciences (AIBS), Athens, Greece.
Petridou ET	Department of Hygiene, Epidemiology and Medical Statistics, Athens University Medical School, Athens, Greece.
Rafailidis PI	Alfa Institute of Biomedical Sciences (AIBS), Athens, Greece.

Hungary

Name of Author	Institutional Affiliation
Hutas G	Semmelweis University, Department of Rheumatology, Polyclinic of the Hospitaller Brothers of St John of God, Budapest, Hungary. gaborhutas@gmail.com

Israel

Name of Author	Institutional Affiliation
Kapelushnik J	Department of Pediatrics, Soroka University Medical Center, Beer Sheva, Israel. shimriti@bgu.ac.il
Nagler A	Division of Hematology and Bone Marrow Transplantation, Chaim Sheba Medical Center, Tel-Hashomer, Israel. ashimoni@sheba.health.gov.il
Shabbat S	Department of Pediatrics, Soroka University Medical Center, Beer Sheva, Israel. shimriti@bgu.ac.il
Shimoni A	Division of Hematology and Bone Marrow Transplantation, Chaim Sheba Medical Center, Tel-Hashomer, Israel. ashimoni@sheba.health.gov.il

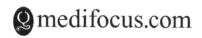
medifocus.com

Slavin S — Institute of Hematology, Tel Hashomer, Israel. arnon.nagler@sheba.health.gov.il

Italy

Name of Author	Institutional Affiliation
Boffetta P	Childhood Cancer Registry of Piedmont, Cancer Epidemiology Unit, CPO Piemonte, CeRMS, University of Turin, Via Santena 7, 10126, Turin, Italy. milena.maule@unito.it
Bosetti C	Istituto di Ricerche Farmacologiche Mario Negri, Milan, Italy. bosetti@marionegri.it
Brugiatelli M	Dipartimento di Oncologia ed Ematologia, Universita di Modena Centro Oncologico Modenese Policlinico, 41100 Modena, Italy. ssacchi@unimo.it
Cavalli F	Unit of Lymphoid Malignancies, San Raffaele Scientific Institute, Milan, Italy. andres.ferreri@hsr.it
Chimienti E	Division of Medical Oncology, National Cancer Institute, Aviano, Italy.
Fabbri A	Unit of Haematology and Transplants, Policlinico S Maria alle Scotte, University of Siena, Siena, Italy. fabbri7@unisi.it
Fanti S	Department of Nuclear Medicine, Institute of Emathology, Policlinico S. Orsola-Malpighi, Bologna, Italy.
Federico M	Dipartimento di Oncologia ed Ematologia, Universita di Modena e Reggio Emilia, Centro Oncologico Modenese, Via del Pozzo, 71 41100, Modena, Italy. federico@unimore.it
Ferreri AJ	Unit of Lymphoid Malignancies, San Raffaele Scientific Institute, Milan, Italy. andres.ferreri@hsr.it
Ferrucci PF	Department of Haematoncology, European Institute of Oncology (IEO), Milan, Italy. pier.ferrucci@ieo.it
La Vecchia C	Istituto di Ricerche Farmacologiche Mario Negri, Milan, Italy.

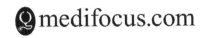

Lauria F	Unit of Haematology and Transplants, Policlinico S Maria alle Scotte, University of Siena, Siena, Italy. fabbri7@unisi.it
Luminari S	Dipartimento di Oncologia ed Ematologia, Universita di Modena e Reggio Emilia, Centro Oncologico Modenese, Via del Pozzo, 71 41100, Modena, Italy. federico@unimore.it
Maule M	Childhood Cancer Registry of Piedmont, Cancer Epidemiology Unit, CPO Piemonte, CeRMS, University of Turin, Via Santena 7, 10126, Turin, Italy. milena.maule@unito.it
Motta G	Department of Internal Medicine, University of Genoa, Room 221, V.le Benedetto XV 6, 16132 Genoa, Italy.
Nencioni A	Department of Internal Medicine, University of Genoa, Room 221, V.le Benedetto XV 6, 16132 Genoa, Italy.
Pirani M	Department of Oncology and Hematology, University of Modena and Reggio Emilia, Modena, Italy.
Re A	Division of Hematology, Spedali Civili di Brescia, Brescia, Italy. sandrore@aruba.it
Rossi G	Division of Hematology, Spedali Civili di Brescia, Brescia, Italy. sandrore@aruba.it
Sacchi S	Dipartimento di Oncologia ed Ematologia, Universita di Modena Centro Oncologico Modenese Policlinico, 41100 Modena, Italy. ssacchi@unimo.it
Scotti L	Istituto di Ricerche Farmacologiche Mario Negri, Milan, Italy.
Tirelli U	Division of Medical Oncology, National Cancer Institute, Aviano, Italy.
Tsamita CS	Department of Nuclear Medicine, Institute of Emathology, Policlinico S. Orsola-Malpighi, Bologna, Italy.
Zucca E	Department of Haematoncology, European Institute of Oncology (IEO), Milan, Italy. pier.ferrucci@ieo.it

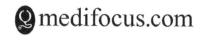

Japan

Name of Author	Institutional Affiliation
Hotta T	Division of Hematology, Department of Internal Medicine, Tokai University, Isehara, Kanagawa, Japan. 8jmmd004@is.icc.u-tokai.ac.jp
Katsuya H	Department of Medical Oncology and Hematology, Fukuoka University Hospital, Fukuoka, Japan.
Nagai H	Clinical Research Center for Blood Diseases, National Hospital Organization Nagoya Medical Center, Nagoya, Japan. tterasawa@tufts-nemc.org
Ohmachi K	Division of Hematology, Department of Internal Medicine, Tokai University, Isehara, Kanagawa, Japan. 8jmmd004@is.icc.u-tokai.ac.jp
Tamura K	Department of Medical Oncology and Hematology, Fukuoka University Hospital, Fukuoka, Japan.
Terasawa T	Clinical Research Center for Blood Diseases, National Hospital Organization Nagoya Medical Center, Nagoya, Japan. tterasawa@tufts-nemc.org
Watanabe T	National Cancer Center Hospital, Hematology Division, 5-1-1, Tsukiji, Chuo-ku, Tokyo 104-0045, Japan. takawata@ncc.go.jp

Korea

Name of Author	Institutional Affiliation
Choi HY	College of Pharmacy, Yeungnam University, Gyeongsan, Kyungbuk, Korea.
Kim JE	Department of Oncology, Asan Medical Center, University of Ulsan College of Medicine, 86 Asan byeongwon-gil, Songpa-gu, 138-736 Seoul, Republic of Korea.
Park BB	Division of Hematology/Oncology, Department of Internal Medicine, Hanyang University College of Medicine, Seoul, South Korea.

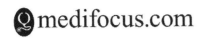

Suh C	Department of Oncology, Laboratory Medicine, and Pathology, Asan Medical Center, University of Ulsan College of Medicine, Seoul, Korea.
Yoo BK	College of Pharmacy, Yeungnam University, Gyeongsan, Kyungbuk, Korea.
Yoon DH	Department of Oncology, Laboratory Medicine, and Pathology, Asan Medical Center, University of Ulsan College of Medicine, Seoul, Korea.

Netherlands

Name of Author	Institutional Affiliation
Brenner H	Comprehensive Cancer Centre South, Eindhoven Cancer Registry, Eindhoven, The Netherlands. research@ikz.nl
Mols F	Comprehensive Cancer Center South, Eindhoven Cancer Registry, Eindhoven, the Netherlands. f.mols@uvt.nl
Oerlemans S	Research Department, Comprehensive Cancer Centre South, Eindhoven, The Netherlands. s.oerlemans@ikz.nl
Schuurmans M	Department of Neuro-Oncology, Daniel den Hoed Cancer Centre, Erasmus MC, Rotterdam, the Netherlands.
van de Poll-Franse LV	Research Department, Comprehensive Cancer Centre South, Eindhoven, The Netherlands. s.oerlemans@ikz.nl
van de Schans SA	Comprehensive Cancer Centre South, Eindhoven Cancer Registry, Eindhoven, The Netherlands. research@ikz.nl
van den Bent MJ	Department of Neuro-Oncology, Daniel den Hoed Cancer Centre, Erasmus MC, Rotterdam, the Netherlands.

New Zealand

Name of Author	Institutional Affiliation
Garnock-Jones KP	Adis, a Wolters Kluwer Business, Auckland, New Zealand. demail@adis.co.nz

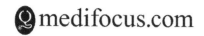 medifocus.com

Nigeria

Name of Author	Institutional Affiliation
Omoti AE	Department of Haematology, University of Benin Teaching Hospital, Benin City, Nigeria. ediomoti@yahoo.com
Omoti CE	Department of Haematology, University of Benin Teaching Hospital, Benin City, Nigeria. ediomoti@yahoo.com

Poland

Name of Author	Institutional Affiliation
Centkowski P	Department of Hematology, Institute of Hematology and Transfusion Medicine, I. Gandhi Street 14, 02776, Warsaw, Poland.
Warzocha K	Department of Hematology, Institute of Hematology and Transfusion Medicine, I. Gandhi Street 14, 02776, Warsaw, Poland.

South Africa

Name of Author	Institutional Affiliation
Novitzky N	University of Cape Town Leukaemia Centre and Department of Haematology, Groote Schuur Hospital, Cape Town, Western Cape, South Africa. novitzky@cormack.uct.ac.za
Thomas V	University of Cape Town Leukaemia Centre and Department of Haematology, Groote Schuur Hospital, Cape Town, Western Cape, South Africa. novitzky@cormack.uct.ac.za

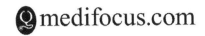

South Korea

Name of Author	Institutional Affiliation
Kim BK	Department of Internal Medicine, Seoul National University College of Medicine, 101 Daehak-ro, Jongro-gu, Seoul, 110-744, South Korea.
Kim JW	Department of Internal Medicine, Seoul National University College of Medicine, 101 Daehak-ro, Jongro-gu, Seoul, 110-744, South Korea.
Suh C	Department of Internal Medicine, Asan Medical Center, University of Ulsan College of Medicine, Songpa-gu, Seoul, South Korea.
Sym SJ	Department of Internal Medicine, Asan Medical Center, University of Ulsan College of Medicine, Songpa-gu, Seoul, South Korea.

Sweden

Name of Author	Institutional Affiliation
Eid JE	Departments of Oncology and Haematology, Karolinska University Hospital, Stockholm, Sweden. anders.osterborg@karolinska.se
Osterborg A	Departments of Oncology and Haematology, Karolinska University Hospital, Stockholm, Sweden. anders.osterborg@karolinska.se

Switzerland

Name of Author	Institutional Affiliation
Cavalli F	Research Division, Oncology Institute of Southern Switzerland, Ospedale San Giovanni, Bellinzona. ielsg@ticino.com
Froesch P	IOSI, Oncology Institute of Southern Switzerland, Bellinzona.
Ozsahin M	Department of Radiation Oncology, Centre Hospitalier Universitaire Vaudois, Lausanne, Switzerland.

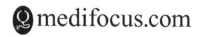

Rossier C	Department of Radiation Oncology, Centre Hospitalier Universitaire Vaudois, Lausanne, Switzerland.
Zucca E	Research Division, Oncology Institute of Southern Switzerland, Ospedale San Giovanni, Bellinzona. ielsg@ticino.com

Taiwan

Name of Author	Institutional Affiliation
Chen PJ	Department of Oncology, National Taiwan University Hospital, Taipei, Taiwan.
Hsu C	Department of Oncology, National Taiwan University Hospital, Taipei, Taiwan.

Turkey

Name of Author	Institutional Affiliation
Abali H	Department of Internal Medicine, Medical Oncology Unit, Mersin University, Mersin, Turkey. habali1970@yahoo.com
Aksakal N	Gazi University Faculty of Medicine, Department of Pediatric Oncology, Ankara, Turkey.
Bora H	Department of Pediatric Oncology, Gazi University Faculty of Medicine, Ankara, Turkey.
Karadeniz C	Gazi University Faculty of Medicine, Department of Pediatric Oncology, Ankara, Turkey.
Oguz A	Department of Pediatric Oncology, Gazi University Faculty of Medicine, Ankara, Turkey.
Zengin N	Department of Internal Medicine, Medical Oncology Unit, Mersin University, Mersin, Turkey. habali1970@yahoo.com

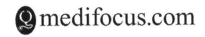

United Kingdom

Name of Author	Institutional Affiliation
Birch JM	University of Manchester and Cancer Research UK, Paediatric and Familial Cancer Research Group, Royal Manchester Children's Hospital, Manchester, United Kingdom. dong.pang@manchester.ac.uk
Bishton MJ	Department of Haematology, Nottingham City Hospital, Nottingham, UK. mj_bishton@hotmail.com
Bloor AJ	Department of Haematology, Royal Free and University College London School of Medicine, London, United Kingdom. drbloor@tiscali.co.uk
El-Helw LM	Weston Park Hospital, YCR Academic Unit of Clinical Oncology, Sheffield, S10 2SJ, UK.
Gribben JG	Barts and The London School of Medicine, London, United Kingdom. j.gribben@qmul.ac.uk
Hancock BW	Royal Hallamshire Hospital, Sheffield, UK.
Haynes AP	Department of Haematology, Nottingham City Hospital, Nottingham, UK. mj_bishton@hotmail.com
Hoskin P	Haematology Trials Group, University College London Cancer Trials Centre, UK.
Illidge TM	University of Manchester, Manchester Academic Health Science Centre, School of Cancer and Enabling Sciences, School of Medicine, Manchester, M20 4BX, UK.
Kane EV	Epidemiology and Genetics Unit, Department of Health Sciences, Seebohm Rowntree Building, University of York, YO10 5DD, UK. eleanor.kane@egu.york.ac.uk <eleanor.kane@egu.york.ac.uk>
Kirby AM	Department of Clinical Oncology, Guy's and St Thomas' NHS Trust, London, UK. annakirby@doctors.org.uk
Lowry L	Haematology Trials Group, University College London Cancer Trials Centre, UK.
Mackinnon S	Department of Haematology, Royal Free and University College London School of Medicine, London, United Kingdom. drbloor@tiscali.co.uk

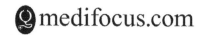

Maloney DG	Barts and The London School of Medicine, London, United Kingdom. j.gribben@qmul.ac.uk
Mayes S	University of Manchester, Manchester Academic Health Science Centre, School of Cancer and Enabling Sciences, School of Medicine, Manchester, M20 4BX, UK.
Mikhaeel NG	Department of Clinical Oncology, Guy's and St Thomas' NHS Trust, London, UK. annakirby@doctors.org.uk
Mukherji D	St Georges Hospital, Blackshaw Road, Tooting, London SW170QT, UK.
Newton R	Epidemiology and Genetics Unit, Department of Health Sciences, Seebohm Rowntree Building, University of York, YO10 5DD, UK. eleanor.kane@egu.york.ac.uk <eleanor.kane@egu.york.ac.uk>
Pang D	University of Manchester and Cancer Research UK, Paediatric and Familial Cancer Research Group, Royal Manchester Children's Hospital, Manchester, United Kingdom. dong.pang@manchester.ac.uk
Pettengell R	St Georges Hospital, Blackshaw Road, Tooting, London SW170QT, UK.
Russell N	Department of Hematology, Nottingham University Hospitals NHS Trust (City Campus), Nottingham NG5 1PB, United Kingdom. nigel.russell@nottingham.ac.uk
Schmitz N	Department of Hematology, Nottingham University Hospitals NHS Trust (City Campus), Nottingham NG5 1PB, United Kingdom. nigel.russell@nottingham.ac.uk
Wright J	Royal Hallamshire Hospital, Sheffield, UK.

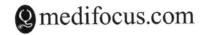

NOTES

Use this page for taking notes as you review your Guidebook

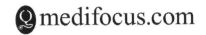 **medifocus.com**

5 - Tips on Finding and Choosing a Doctor

Introduction

One of the most important decisions confronting patients who have been diagnosed with a serious medical condition is finding and choosing a qualified physician who will deliver a high level and quality of medical care in accordance with currently accepted guidelines and standards of care. Finding the "best" doctor to manage your condition, however, can be a frustrating and time-consuming experience unless you know what you are looking for and how to go about finding it.

The process of finding and choosing a physician to manage your specific illness or condition is, in some respects, analogous to the process of making a decision about whether or not to invest in a particular stock or mutual fund. After all, you wouldn't invest your hard eared money in a stock or mutual fund without first doing exhaustive research about the stock or fund's past performance, current financial status, and projected future earnings. More than likely you would spend a considerable amount of time and energy doing your own research and consulting with your stock broker before making an informed decision about investing. The same general principle applies to the process of finding and choosing a physician. Although the process requires a considerable investment in terms of both time and energy, the potential payoff can be well worth it--after all, what can be more important than your health and well-being?

This section of your Guidebook offers important tips for how to find physicians as well as suggestions for how to make informed choices about choosing a doctor who is right for you.

Tips for Finding Physicians

Finding a highly qualified, competent, and compassionate physician to manage your specific illness or condition takes a lot of hard work and energy but is an investment that is well-worth the effort. It is important to keep in mind that you are not looking for just any general physician but rather for a physician who has expertise in the treatment and management of your specific illness or condition. Here are some suggestions for where you can turn to identify and locate physicians who specialize in managing your disorder:

- **Your Doctor** - Your family physician (family medicine or internal medicine specialist) is a good starting point for finding a physician who specializes in your illness. Chances are that your doctor already knows several specialists in your geographic area who specialize in your illness and can recommend several names to you. Your doctor can also provide you with information about their qualifications, training, and hospital affiliations.

- **Your Peer Network** - Your family, friends, and co-workers can be a potentially very useful network for helping you find a physician who specializes in your illness. They may know someone else with this condition and may be able to put you in touch with them to find out which doctors they can recommend. If you have friends, neighbors, or relatives who work in hospitals (e.g., nurses, social workers, administrators), they may be a potentially valuable source for helping you find a physician who specializes in your condition.

- **Hospitals and Medical Centers** - Hospitals and medical centers are, potentially, an excellent source for finding physicians who specialize in treating specific diseases. Simply contact hospitals and major medical centers in your city, county, or state and ask if they have anyone on their staff who specializes in treating your condition. When you call, ask to speak to someone in the specific Department that cares for patients with the illness. For example, if you have been diagnosed with cancer, ask to speak with someone in the Department of Hematology and Oncology. If you are not sure which Department treats patients with your specific condition, ask to speak to someone in the Department of Medicine since this Department is the umbrella for many other medical specialties.

- **Organizations and Support Groups** - Many disease organizations and support groups that cater to patients with a specific illness or condition maintain physician referral lists and may be able to recommend doctors in your geographic area who specialize in the treatment and management of your specific disorder. This *MediFocus Guidebook* includes a select listing of disease organizations and support groups that you may wish to contact to ask for a physician referral.

- **Managed Care Plans** - If you belong to a managed care plan, you can obtain a list of physicians who belong to the Plan from the plan's membership services office. Keep in mind, however, that your choices will usually be limited to only those doctors who belong to the Plan. If you decide to go outside the Plan, you will likely have to pay for the doctor's services "out of pocket".

- **Medical Journals** - Many doctors based at major medical centers and universities who have special interest in a particular disease or condition conduct research and publish their findings in leading medical journals. Searching the medical literature can help you identify and locate leading physicians who are recognized as experts in their field about a particular illness. This *MediFocus Guidebook* includes an extensive listing of the names and institutional affiliations of physicians and researchers, in the United States and other countries, who have recently published their studies about this specific medical condition in leading medical journals. You can also conduct your own online search for your illness or condition and identify additional authors and hospitals who specialize in the disease using the PubMed database available at http://www.nlm.nih.gov.

- **American Medical Association** - The American Medical Association (AMA) is the nation's largest professional medical association that represents many doctors in the United States and also provides a free physician locator service called "AMA Physician Select" available at http://dbapps.ama-assn.org/aps/amahg.htm. You can search the AMA database by either "Physician Name" or "Medical Specialty". You can find information about physicians including medical school and residency training, area of specialty, and contact information.

- **American Board of Medical Specialists** - The American Board of Medical Specialists (ABMS) publishes a geographical list of board-certified physicians called the Official ABMS Directory of Board Certified Medical Specialists that is available in most public libraries. Physicians who are listed in the ABMS Directory are board-certified in a medical specialty meaning that they have passed rigorous certification examinations administered by a board of medical specialists. There are 24 specialty boards that are recognized by the ABMS and the AMA. Each candidate applying for board certification must pass a written examination given by the specific specialty board and 15 of the specialty boards also require candidates to pass an oral examination in order to obtain board certification. To find out if a particular physician you are considering is board certified:

  - Visit your local public library and ask for a copy of the Official ABMS Directory of Board Certified Medical Specialists.

  - Search the ABMS web site at http://www.abms.org/login.asp.

  - Call the ABMS toll free at 1-866-275-2267.

- **American Society of Clinical Oncology** - The American Society of Clinical Onclology (ASC)) is the largest professional organization that represents physicians who specialize in treating cancer patients (oncologists). The ASCO provides a searchable database of ASCO members called "Find an Oncologist" that you can access online at http://www.asco.org. You can search the "Find an Oncologist" database for a cancer specialist by name, city, state, country, or specialty area.

- **American Cancer Society** - The American Cancer Society (ACS) is a nationwide voluntary health organization dedicated to helping cancer patients and survivors through research, education, advocacy, and services. The ACS web site http://www.cancer.org is not only an excellent resource for cancer information but also includes a "Message Board" where you can ask questions, exchange ideas, and share stories. The ACS Message Board is also a potentially useful source for locating an oncologist in your geographical area who specializes in your specific type of cancer. You can also contact the ACS toll free by calling 1-800-ACS-2345.

- **National Comprehensive Cancer Network** - The National Comprehensive Cancer Network (NCCN) is an alliance of 19 of the world's leading cancer centers and is dedicated to helping patients and health care professionals make informed decisions about cancer care. You can find a listing of the 19 NCCN member cancer institutions on the NCCN web site at http://www.nccn.org/. You can also search the NCCN "Physician Directory" for doctors located at any of the 19 NCCN member cancer institutions at http://www.nccn.org/physician_directory/SearchPers.asp. This database is an excellent resource for locating leading cancer specialists nationwide who specialize in your specific type of cancer.

- **National Cancer Institute Clinical Trials Database** - The National Cancer Institute (NCI) is part of the National Institutes of Health (NIH) and coordinates the National Cancer Program which conducts and supports research, training, and a variety of other programs dedicated to prevention and treatment of cancer. The NCI maintains an extensive cancer clinical trials database that you can access at http://www.cancer.gov/clinicaltrials. You can search the database for current clinical trials by type of cancer and even limit your search to clinical trials within you geographical area by putting in your Zip Code. The NCI clinical trials database also provides contact information for the physicians who serve as the study coordinators for each clinical trial. This database is a valuable resource for identifying and locating leading physicians in your local area and around the country who are conducting cutting-edge clinical research about your specific type of cancer.

- **National Center for Complementary and Alternative Medicine** - The National Center for Complementary and Alternative Medicine (NCCAM) is part of the National Institutes of Health (NIH) and is dedicated to exploring complementary and alternative medicine healing practices in the context of rigorous scientific research and methodology. The NCCAM web site http://nccam.nih.gov/ includes publications, frequently asked questions, and useful links to other complementary and alternative medicine resources. If you have questions about complementary and alternative medicine practices for your particular illness or medical condition, you can contact

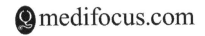

the NCCAM Clearinghouse toll-free in the U.S. at 1-888-644-6226 or 301-519-3153. You can also contact the NCCAM Clearinghouse by E-mail: info@nccam.nih.gov.

- **National Organization for Rare Disorders** - The National Organization for Rare Disorders (NORD) is a federation of voluntary health organizations dedicated to helping patients with rare "orphan" diseases and their families. There are over 6,000 rare or "orphan" diseases that are estimated to affect approximately 25 million Americans. You can search NORD's "Rare Diseases Database" for information about rare diseases at http://www.rarediseases.org/search/rdblist.html. In addition to providing useful information about rare diseases, NORD maintains a confidential "Networking Program" for its members to enable them to communicate with other patients who suffer from the same disorder. To learn more about NORD's Networking Program, you can send an E mail to: orphan@rarediseases.org.

How to Make Informed Choices About Physicians

It has generally been assumed by many people that the longer a physician has been in practice, the more experience, knowledge, and skills he/she has accumulated and, therefore, the higher the quality of care they provide to their patients. Recent research conducted by a group of doctors from the Harvard Medical School, however, seems to strongly suggest that this premise may not be true. In an article published in February 2005 in the *Annals of Internal Medicine* (Volume 142, No. 4, pp. 260-303), the Harvard researchers seriously challenged the common assumption that the more clinical experience a physician has accumulated, the higher the level of medical care they provide to their patients.

In fact, surprisingly, the researchers found an inverse (opposite) relationship between the number of years that a physician has been in practice (i.e., experience) and the quality of care that the physician provides. In other words, the widely held belief that "practice makes perfect" does not necessarily apply to all physicians and should not be the sole criteria used by patients in their decision analysis for choosing a physician. The underlying message of this study is that the length of time a physician has been in practice does not necessarily equate to a high quality of medical care unless the doctor takes steps to keep abreast with new advances and changing patterns of clinical practice.

Here are some important issues you need to consider and carefully research before making an informed decision about choosing your doctor:

- **Board Certification** - Board certified doctors are required to have extra training after medical school to become specialists in a particular field of medicine and are required to take continuing education courses in order to maintain their board certification status. Check with the American Board of Medical Specialists (ABMS) to determine if a specific physician you are considering is board certified in a particular medical specialty. To find out if a particular physician you are considering is board certified:

  - Visit your local public library and ask for a copy of the Official ABMS Directory of Board Certified Medical Specialists.

  - Search the ABMS web site at http://www.abms.org/login.asp.

  - Call the ABMS toll free at 1-866-275-2267.

- **Experience** - As noted above, research from the Harvard Medical School strongly suggests that how long a physician has been in practice (i.e., experience) does not necessarily correlate with a high level of medical care. The most important issue, therefore, is not how long a doctor has been in practice but rather how much experience the physician has in treating your specific illness or medical condition. Some physicians who have been in practice for many decades may have only treated a small number of patients with the specific disorder, whereas, some younger physicians who have been in practice only a few years may have already treated hundreds of patients with the same disorder. Here are some suggestions for helping you find out about a particular physician's experience in treating your specific illness:

  - Call the physician's office and speak with a staff member such as a nurse or physician's assistant. Ask them for information about how many patients with your specific medical condition the physician treats during the course of a year. Ask how many patients with this condition the physician is currently treating. You will have to call several different physicians' offices in order to have a basis for comparing the numbers of patients.

  - Find out if the physician has published any articles about the condition in reputable medical journals by doing an author search online. You can conduct an online author search using PubMed at http://www.nlm.nih.gov. Simply click on the "PubMed" icon, select the "author" field from the "Limits" menu, enter the physician's name (last name followed by first initial), and then click on the "Go" button. The author search will retrieve all articles published by the particular physician you are considering.

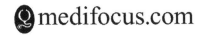

- Talk with your family physician and ask if he/she can provide you with any information about the particular physician's experience in treating patients with your specific illness or condition.

- Contact disease organizations and support groups that specialize in helping patients with your specific disorder and ask if they can provide you with any information, including experience, about the physician you are considering.

- **Medical School Affiliation** - Find out if the physician you are considering also has a joint faculty appointment at a medical school. In general, practicing community physicians with a joint academic appointment at a medical school are more likely to be in contact with leading medical experts and may be more up-to-date with the latest advances in research and treatments than community based physicians who are not affiliated with a medical school.

- **Hospital Affiliation** - Find out about the hospitals that the doctor uses. In the event that you need to be treated at a hospital, is the hospital where the physician has admitting privileges nearby to your home or will you (and your family members) have to travel a considerable distance?

- **Hospital Accreditation** - Find out if the hospital where the physician has admitting privileges is accredited by the Joint Commission on Accreditation of Healthcare Organizations (JCAHO). You can find information about a specific hospital's accreditation status by searching the JCAHO web site at http://www.jointcommission.org/. The JCAHO is an independent, not-for-profit organization that evaluates and accredits more than 15,000 health care organizations and programs in the United States. To receive and maintain JCAHO accreditation, a health care organization must undergo an on-site survey by a JCAHO survey team at least every three years and meet specific standards and performance measurements that affect the safety and quality of patient care.

- **Health Insurance Coverage** - Find out if the physician is covered by your health insurance plan. If you belong to a managed care plan (HMO or PPO), you are usually restricted to using specific physicians who also belong to the Plan. If you decide to use a physician who is "outside the network," you will likely have to pay "out of pocket" for the services provided.

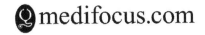 medifocus.com

NOTES

Use this page for taking notes as you review your Guidebook

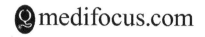

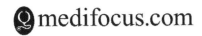

6 - Directory of Organizations

American Cancer Society
1599 Clifton Road NE; Atlanta, GA 30329-4251
800.227.2345; 404.486.0100
www.cancer.org

American Institute for Cancer Research; Nutrition Hotline
1759 R St. NW; Washington, DC 20009
800.843.8114; 202.328.7744
www.aicr.org

American Society of Pediatric Hematology/Oncology
4700 West Lake; Glenview, IL 60025-1485
847.375.4716
info@aspho.org
www.aspho.org

Association of Cancer Online Resources
www.acor.org

Cancer Care
275 Seventh Avenue; New York, NY 10001
800.813.4673; 212.712.8400
info@cancercare.org
www.cancercare.org

Cancer Caring Center
4117 Liberty Avenue; Pittsburgh, PA 15224
412.622.1212
info@cancercaring.org
www.cancercaring.org

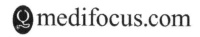

Cancer Hope Network
2 North Road; Chester, NJ 07930
877.467.3638; 908.879.4039
info@cancerhopenetwork.org
www.cancerhopenetwork.org

Cancer Information Service; National Cancer Institute
6116 Executive Boulevard; Room 3036A; Bethesda, MD 20892
800.422.6237   800.332.8615 (TTY)
www.cancer.gov

CancerHelp (UK)
0808 800 40 40
www.cancerhelp.org.uk

Candlelighters Childhood Cancer Foundation
POB 498; Kensington, MD 20895
800.366.2223;   301.962.3520
staff@candlelighters.org
www.candlelighters.org

Center for International Bone & Marrow Transplant Research
9200 W. Wisconsin Avenue Suite C5500 Milwaukee, WI 53226
414.805.0700
cibmtr-contact@nmdp.org
www.cibmtr.org

Children's Cancer and Blood Foundation
333 East 38th Street, Suite 830, New York, New York 10016
212.297.4336
www.childrenscbf.org

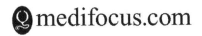

Cleveland Clinic Taussig Cancer Center
9500 Euclid Avenue; Cleveland, OH 44195
800.862.7798   800.223.2273
www.clevelandclinic.org/cancer

Cure Search; Childrens Oncology Group
4600 East-West Highway; Suite 600; Bethesda, MD 20814-3457
800.458.6223;   240.235.2200
info@curesearch.org
www.curesearch.org

Dana Farber Cancer Institute
44 Binney Street; Boston, MA 02115
866.408.3324;   617.632.5330 (TDD)
www.dana-farber.org

Duke University Medical Center
Erwin Road Durham, NC 27710
(919) 684-8111
www.mc.duke.edu

European Organization for Research and Treatment of Cancer
Avenue E Mounier 83, boite 11; B-1200, Brussels; BELGIUM
+32 2-774-1611
www.eortc.org

Fox Chase Cancer Center
33 Cottman Avenue; Philadelphia, PA 19111
888.369.2427   215.728.6900
www.fccc.edu

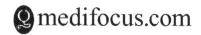

H. Lee Moffitt Cancer Center and Research Institute
12902 Magnolia Drive Tampa, FL 33612
(813) 972-4673
www.moffitt.usf.edu

Hospital of the University of Pennsylvania
3400 Spruce Street Philadelphia, PA 19104
(215) 662-4000
www.pennhealth.com

Johns Hopkins Hospital
600 North Wolfe Street Baltimore, MD 21287
(410) 955-5000
www.hopkinsmedicine.org

Leukemia and Lymphoma Society
1311 Mamaroneck Avenue; White Plains, NY 10605
800.955.4572; 914.949.5213
www.leukemia-lymphoma.org

Look Good...Feel Better; American Cancer Society
1599 Clifton Road, NE; Atlanta, GA 30329
800.395.5665
www.lookgoodfeelbetter.org

Lymphoma Foundation of Canada
16-1375 Southdown Road; Suite 236; Mississauga, Ontario; L5J 2Z1 CANADA
866.659.5556; 905.822.5135
info@lymphoma.ca
www.lymphoma.ca

Lymphoma Information Network
info@lymphomainfo.net.
www.lymphomainfo.net

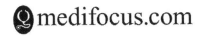

Lymphoma Research Foundation
8800 Venice Boulevard; Suite 207; Los Angeles, CA 90034
800.500.9976; 310.204.7040
helpline@lymphoma.org
www.lymphoma.org

M.D. Anderson Cancer Center
1515 Holcombe Blvd.; Houston, TX 77030
800.392.1611 713.792.3245; 713.792.6161 (fax)
www.mdanderson.org

Macmillan Cancer Support; Cancer Bacup
89 Albert Embankment London SE1 7UQ UK
020 7840 7840
www.cancerbacup.org.uk

Massachusetts General Hospital
55 Fruit Street Boston, MA 02114
(617) 726-2000
www.massgeneral.org

Mayo Clinic
1216 Second Street SW Rochester, MN 55902
(507) 255-5123
www.mayoclinic.org

Memorial Sloan-Kettering Cancer Center
1275 York Avenue; New York, NY 10021
800.525.2225 212.639.2000
www.mskcc.org

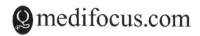

National Bone Marrow Transplant Link

20411 West Twelve Mile Road; Suite 108; Southfield, MI 48076
800.546.5268;   248.358.1886
www.nbmtlink.org

National Comprehensive Cancer Network

275 Commerce Dr, Suite 300 Fort Washington, PA 19034
215.690.0300
www.nccn.org

National Marrow Donor Program.

3001 Broadway Street NE; Suite 500; Minneapolis, MN 55413
800.627.7692   612.627.5800
www.marrow.org

Ohio State University James Cancer Hospital

370 West 9th Avenue Columbus, OH 43210
(614) 293-8000
www.osumedcenter.edu

People Living with Cancer; American Society of Clinical Oncology

2318 Mill Road, Suite 800, Alexandria, VA 22314
571-483-1780;   888-651-3038
contactus@cancer.net
www.cancer.net

Ronald Reagan UCLA Medical Center

10833 Le Conte Avenue Los Angeles, CA 90095
(310) 825-9111
www.uclahealth.org

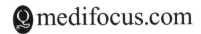

Stanford Hospital and Clinics

300 Pasteur Drive Palo Alto, CA 94304
(650) 723-4000
www.stanfordhospital.com/

The Cancer Project; Cancer and Nutrition

5100 Wisconsin Avenue Suite 400 Washington, DC 20016
202.244.5038
www.cancerproject.org

The Lymphoma Association (UK)

POB 386; Aylesbury, Bucks HP20 2GA   UK
Helpline: 08 08 808 5555; 01 296 619 400
information@lymphoma.org.uk
www.lymphoma.org.uk

The Wellness Community

919 18th Street NW; Suite 54; Washington, DC 20006
888.793.9355;   202.659.9705
help@thewellnesscommunity.org
www.thewellnesscommunity.org

University of Alabama Hospital at Birmingham

619 South 19th Street Birmingham, AL 35233
(205) 934-4011
www.health.uab.edu

University of California, San Francisco Medical Center

500 Parnassus Avenue San Francisco, CA 94143
(415) 476-1000
www.ucsfhealth.org

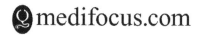

University of Chicago; Cancer Research Center

5841 South Maryland Avenue; Chicago, IL 60637
877.824.0660   773.702.1000
uchospitals.edu/specialties/cancer

University of Michigan Hospitals and Health Centers

1500 East Medical Center Drive Ann Arbor, MI 48109
(734) 936-4000
www.med.umich.edu

University of Southern California; USC/Norris Cancer Center

1441 Eastlake Avenue; Los Angeles, CA 90033
323.865.3000
ccnt.hsc.usc.edu

University of Washington Medical Center

1959 NE Pacific St, Box 356151 Seattle, WA 98195
(206) 598-3300
www.uwmedicine.org/Facilities/UWMedicalCenter/

Vanderbilt University Medical Center

1211 22nd Avenue South Nashville, TN 37232
(615) 322-5000
www.mc.vanderbilt.edu

Women's Cancer Resource Center

5741 Telegraph Avenue; Oakland, CA 94609
888.421.7900; 510.420.7900
wcrc@wcrc.org
www.wcrc.org

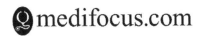 medifocus.com

Complementary and Alternative Medicine Resources

American Academy of Medical Acupuncture
170 East Grand Avenue Suite 330 El Segundo, CA 90245 Phone: 310.364.0193
administrato@medicalacupuncture.org
http://www.medicalacupuncture.org

American Association for Acupuncture and Oriental Medicine
1925 West County Road B2
Roseville, MN 55113
Phone: 651.631.0216
http://www.aaaom.edu

American Association of Naturopathic Physicians
4435 Wisconsin Avenue
Suite 403 Washington, DC 20016
Phone (Toll free): 866.538.2267
Phone: 202.237.8150
http://www.naturopathic.org

American Chiropractic Association
1701 Clarendon Blvd.
Arlington, VA 22209
Phone: 703.276.8800 memberinfo@acatoday.org http://www.amerchiro.org

American Holistic Medical Association
23366 Commerce Park Suite 101B Beachwood, OH 44122 Phone: 216.292.6644
info@holisticmedicine.org http://www.holisticmedicine.org

American Massage Therapy Association
500 Davis Street, Suite 900
Evanston, IL 60201-4695
Phone (Toll-Free): 877.905.2700
Phone: 847.864.0123 info@amtamassage.org http://www.amtamassage.org

National Center for Complementary and Alternative Medicine (NCCAM) Clearinghouse
9000 Rockville Pike Bethesda, MD 20892 Phone: 888.644.6226 info@nccam.nih.gov

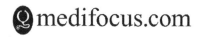

http://nccam.nih.gov

National Center for Homeopathy
801 North Fairfax Street, Suite 306
Alexandria, VA 22314
Phone: 703.548.7790
http://www.homeopathic.org

Office of Dietary Supplements, National Institutes of Health
6100 Executive Boulevard
Room 3B01, MSC 7517
Bethesda, MD 20892-7517
Phone: 301.435.2920 ods@nih.gov http://ods.od.nih.gov

Rosenthal Center for Complementary and Alternative Medicine
Columbia Presbyterian Hospital
630 West 168th Street
Box 75
New York, NY 10032
Phone: 212.342.0101
http://rosenthal.hs.columbia.edu

12023896R00107

Made in the USA
Charleston, SC
06 April 2012